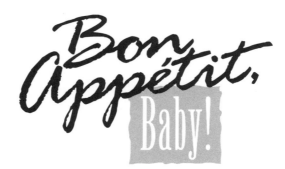

Your Breastfeeding Guide

Elaine Moran

D1307739

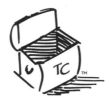

Treasured Child Publications
Freedom, California

Published by Treasured Child Publications, P.O. Box 656, Freedom, California 95019-0656

Cover art and line art by Kimball Barton
Illustrations by Candace Wright and Cindy Davis
Text design and layout by Slub Design

ISBN 978-0-9674315-1-2

This book is available at quantity discounts. For pricing and ordering information contact:

Treasured Child Publications
P.O. Box 656
Freedom, California 95019-0656
Phone: 1-888-942-7894 (toll-free)
Fax: 1-415-723-7618
Email: info@bonappetitbaby.com

Visit our Website at: www.BonAppetitBaby.com

Disclaimer: The information contained in this book is general information and the suggestions, procedures, and/or materials are not intended as medical advice or as a substitute for a consultation with your health care provider. Medical supervision is recommended for prenatal and postnatal care and any other matters concerning your health. Individual questions should be addressed to your health care provider, lactation specialist, or registered dietitian. Do not start any diet or exercise program without consulting your health care provider. Treasured Child Publications disclaims all responsibility arising from any adverse effects or results that occur as a result of the application of the information contained in this book.

First printing, January 2005
Reprinted, January 2011
10 9 8 7 6 5 4 3 2

Printed in Singapore by Craft Print International Ltd.

*This book is dedicated
to all mothers, everywhere,
for your courage and strength.*

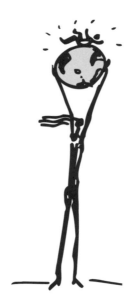

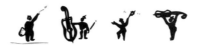

Author's Note:

For the ease of reading, I have chosen to use the male gender throughout this book when referring to the baby.

Contents

Introduction 1

Breastfeeding Benefits Chart 2

CHAPTER 1: Is Breastfeeding For You? 3

Who Can Breastfeed? 3
Commonly Asked Questions About Breastfeeding 3
Why Is Breastfeeding So Important? 11
What Can I Expect as a Breastfeeding Mother? 13
What Can I Expect as a Breastfeeding Father? 14

CHAPTER 2: Breastfeeding Basics 17

Preparing For Breastfeeding 17
How Breastfeeding Works 19
Arriving at the Hospital 21
"Breastfeeding Baby In Training" Sign 23
At Home With Your Baby 31
Keeping Track of Your Breastfeeding Baby 37
Baby's Feeding and Diaper Log 38
Breastfeeding and Sexuality 41
Breastfeeding in Public 41

CHAPTER 3: Solving Breastfeeding Problems 45

Identifying Common Newborn Problems 45
Managing Difficulties the Mother May Have 51
Breastfeeding 911: Getting Help 57

CHAPTER 4: Special Situations 63

Breastfeeding After a Cesarean 63
Breastfeeding the Premature Baby 63
Breastfeeding Multiples 64

CHAPTER 5: Adjusting to Motherhood 65

Physical Changes 65
Emotional Changes 66
Relationship Changes 67

CHAPTER 6: Nutrition For the Nursing Mother 69

Breastfeeding Nutrition 69
Breastfeeding and Weight Loss 69
Daily Calorie Requirement 70
The USDA Food Guide Pyramid 71
The U.S. Food Exchange System 71
Your Daily Food Group Servings 72
Food Exchange Lists 72
Fast Foods the Healthy Way 80
Sample Menu 80
Foods That Can Sometimes Cause a Reaction 81
Exercise 82
The Nursing Mother's Daily Nutrition Checklist 83

CHAPTER 7: Starting Solid Foods and Weaning 91

When to Start Solid Foods 91
Suggestions for Weaning 92

CHAPTER 8: Working and Breastfeeding 93

Planning Ahead 93
Returning to Work 95
Expressing Breast Milk 95
Storing Breast Milk 97

The New Mother's Journal 99

Baby's Birth Record. 100
Childbirth Experience 101
Idea Starters 104

Where to Find Help. 112

Index 114

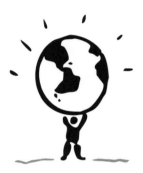

Introduction

Breastfeeding is the way women have fed their babies since the beginning of time—our survival as a species has depended on it. Not long ago, breastfeeding was the *only* way to feed a baby. In many traditional cultures around the world it is still the way of life and a girl grows up seeing her mother, older sisters, aunts, and neighbors breastfeeding their babies. She learns from them how to position her own baby at the breast and tell if he is latched on correctly and getting enough milk.

But because modern man has tried to improve upon nature by inventing infant formula, the tradition of breastfeeding in America has been lost, and the chain of breastfeeding knowledge has been broken. For this reason, it is completely normal if you never thought about breastfeeding before you became pregnant, and you don't know very much about it. Chances are you may have never seen a mother nursing her baby. So even though breastfeeding is a natural thing to do, you may need some help getting started. And like anything else, it takes time, practice, and patience to learn something new—but learning to breastfeed is well worth the effort.

The goal of this book is to show you how breastfeeding will make a difference, not only in your baby's life, but in your life, your family's life, and in society. This book will explain why breastfeeding is so important and show you step-by-step how to nurse your baby. My hope is that once you learn more about breastfeeding and understand its many benefits, you will be convinced that it is the healthiest way to feed your baby.

Many women decide not to breastfeed, or give up early, for many different reasons. In this book, I have tried to offer solutions to some of the most common challenges new mothers face. But no matter how you choose to feed your baby, remember the decision is always yours. Learn everything you can about breastfeeding and parenting, but trust your own instincts—nobody knows better than you what feels right and what is best for you and your baby. You may have already decided to breastfeed, but if you haven't, my hope is that you will at least give breastfeeding a try. Because even if you breastfeed for just one day, one week, or one month, as you will see in the pages that follow, your baby *can* and *will* benefit from it.

I named this book *Bon Appétit, Baby! Your Breastfeeding Guide* because *bon appétit* is a French expression that means "enjoy your meal"—and that is my wish for your baby each time he nurses.

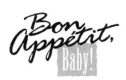

Breastfeeding Benefits Chart

FOR BABY

HEALTH

- stronger immune system
- fewer ear infections
- fewer colds & viruses
- fewer tummy aches
- fewer allergies
- less diaper rash & eczema
- less diarrhea & constipation
- less spitting up & vomiting
- less likely to die of SIDS
- fewer respiratory tract infections
- faster recovery from illnesses
- fewer illnesses, doctor visits, and hospitalizations

NUTRITION AND GROWTH

- the perfect food for babies
- contains all necessary nutrients
- easier to digest than formula
- breast milk changes as baby grows
- premature babies do better
- helps baby's brain develop
- breastfed children have higher IQs
- reduces risk of obesity
- reduces risk of diabetes
- reduces risk of childhood cancers
- reduces risk of asthma
- reduces risk of gastrointestinal infections
- stronger and straighter teeth

BONDING

- creates a strong mother and child bond
- easier to comfort baby when hurt or ill
- satisfies baby's need for closeness and security

FOR MOTHER

PHYSICAL

- aids in natural weight loss
- reduces risk of breast cancer
- reduces risk of ovarian cancer
- reduces risk of cervical cancer
- reduces risk of osteoporosis
- helps uterus return to its normal size sooner
- less postpartum bleeding
- less risk of pregnancy
- makes nighttime feedings easier

EMOTIONAL

- ensures close physical contact
- relaxes the mother
- able to comfort baby quickly
- able to get more rest
- increases self-confidence

FOR FAMILY

- saves time , energy, and money—it's free!
- no bottles to prepare—especially in the middle of the night
- no baby food needed for the first 6 months
- always available, warm, fresh, and sterile
- breast milk doesn't stain
- baby's spit up & stools have less odor
- baby has softer skin and a sweeter smell
- fewer doctor bills
- less missed days of work

FOR SOCIETY

- good for the environment—it conserves energy and produces less solid waste
- cuts down on national health care costs
- contributes to a more productive workforce
- creates a stronger and healthier society

CHAPTER 1

Is Breastfeeding For You?

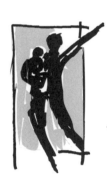

If there were a vaccine you could give your baby that would lessen or prevent a variety of childhood illnesses, help him be healthier, smarter, and more secure, and if it were absolutely free and completely safe, wouldn't you want to know more about it? You probably would, because if you are like most mothers, you want the very best for your baby. And, as you can see from the chart on the opposite page, breastfeeding can do all this—and more! Because of these benefits, The American Academy of Pediatrics (AAP) and the World Health Organization (WHO), along with many other experts around the world, promote breastfeeding as the best way to feed your baby.

Who Can Breastfeed?

No matter what your age, where you live, what kinds of food you eat, what size your breasts, or how calm or nervous you feel in the beginning, **almost any woman can breastfeed**. Even with all the unfairness in the world, Mother Nature has given every new mother an equal chance to give her baby the same best start in life. Believe it or not, this is what our breasts are for!

Although most women are able to breastfeed, there are still a few situations in which mothers cannot nurse their babies. If a mother has a very serious health problem, breastfeeding may not be recommended. A women should **not** breastfeed if she:

- takes street drugs or does not control her alcohol use
- has an infant with galactosemia (an inherited metabolic disorder)
- is infected with HIV (the virus that causes AIDS)
- has active, untreated tuberculosis
- is undergoing treatment for breast cancer

Other conditions such as herpes, hepatitis, and varicella may also affect a mother's ability to nurse. If you have questions about your health and whether you are able to breastfeed, check with your doctor or a lactation specialist who can answer your specific questions.

Commonly Asked Questions About Breastfeeding

There are so many myths about breastfeeding in our culture, and now that you are expecting a baby you may have even heard a few yourself. Sadly, many women don't even try to nurse their babies, or they give up too soon because they have been given poor or incorrect advice from friends, relatives, and even their doctors about breastfeeding. Unfortunately, medical schools don't teach very much on the subject. But more and more, doctors are realizing its importance and are learning more about it. As an expectant mother deciding how to feed your baby, you probably have many questions. The following are answers to some of the most commonly asked questions about breastfeeding to help you separate fact from fiction.

1. Isn't formula just as good as breast milk?

Many modern Americans believe that infant formula is just as good as breast milk, and with all the advertising and marketing by formula companies, maybe you do too. Just a generation ago it was believed that formula feeding was a healthier and more modern way to feed babies. But in recent years, researchers have been seriously studying breast milk and putting formula to the test. Their findings have shown that formula isn't at all what it was cracked up to be—and breastfeeding has now been proven to be the healthiest way to feed babies. **What scientists have discovered is that it is *impossible* to make an infant formula that exactly matches human breast milk.** Your breast milk is custom made for your baby each time he nurses to provide him with the perfect combination of proteins, fats, carbohydrates, and other beneficial ingredients at the exact time he needs it. The makeup of your breast milk changes from day to day to meet your baby's grow-

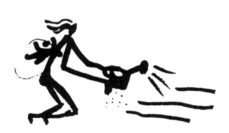

ing needs. Although infant formulas contain many of the same ingredients as breast milk, they are not in the same amounts, they do not change from day to day, and they are not absorbed as efficiently. In addition, breast milk contains *antibodies* (protein molecules) and living white blood cells that fight off infections and diseases and help protect your baby until his immune system is fully developed. These important ingredients can ***never*** be found in an artificial white powder or liquid with an "expiration date." There are also ingredients in breast milk that scientists have not yet identified. Whenever a new ingredient in breast milk is discovered, formula manufacturers scramble to see if they can improve their product to more closely match human breast milk. While infant formulas are an acceptable substitute for those mothers who cannot or choose not to breastfeed, breast milk is unique and superior to any infant formula—and impossible to match exactly, no matter how many times a product is improved upon. If you choose to breastfeed, you can be sure that all the necessary ingredients will always be present in the right amounts to give your baby the healthiest possible start in life.

2. Will breastfeeding hurt?

When you think about breastfeeding, it is normal to wonder if it will be painful. Although there may be some discomfort in the beginning, **breastfeeding should not hurt**. You may have some nipple tenderness during the first few days, which is common, but this should only be temporary as your breasts go through a period of conditioning. Your breasts and nipples are designed to deliver milk to your baby and you should never have pain so badly that you don't want to nurse. When your baby is latched on properly and breastfeeding well, it should feel comfortable and calming for both of you. **If you** are having pain, it is almost always because your baby is not latched on correctly. To reduce soreness, make sure your baby's mouth is wide open and he has the nipple and a good portion of the *areola* (the brown area around your nipple) as far back in his mouth as possible. Your baby should not suck *only* on the nipple. If he is not latched on correctly, break the baby's suction to your breast by gently putting your finger into the corner of his mouth, and then reposition him. See "Latch-on" on PAGE 25 to learn how to get your baby to latch on properly. If breastfeeding becomes painful at any time, get help from your doctor or a lactation specialist.

3. Won't breastfeeding be embarrassing?

It is natural to think that breastfeeding in public or around family and friends might be a little embarrassing—but it doesn't have to be. When babies are hungry, they need to eat just like everyone else. With a little planning and practice you will soon be able to breastfeed anytime, anywhere—and most people won't even know you are feeding your baby! See the section "Breastfeeding in Public" on PAGE 41 for some practical tips on how to breastfeed *discreetly* (without anyone knowing). If it makes you feel more comfortable, you can offer your baby a bottle of expressed breast milk in places where you may be too shy to nurse. Unfortunately, people's lack of understanding has made mothers feel self-conscious about breastfeeding in public places. But times are changing and many states have even passed laws that give mothers the right to breastfeed in public. Remember, breastfeeding is a natural part of being a mother. Be proud that you are giving your baby the very best!

4. Will breastfeeding tie me down?

It takes time and patience to feed a baby no matter which method you choose. Although breastfed babies do need to eat more often than formula-fed babies, breast milk can be more convenient no matter where you are. It is always ready and at the right temperature—your baby is all you need. With formula, you have to fuss with bottles, water, and other feeding equipment, as well as mixing, warming, and chilling the formula. With breastfeeding, your milk is ready the minute your baby is hungry. After the first few weeks, when you have a good milk supply, there is no reason why you can't go out and leave your baby with a family member or babysitter. You can pump your breast milk beforehand and leave it for the caregiver to feed your baby while you are away. See "Expressing Breast Milk" on PAGE 95 for more information.

5. Will breastfeeding spoil my baby?

While you are pregnant, your baby is being nourished and comforted inside your womb—24 hours a day. He hears your heartbeat and feels the warmth and security of your body. After birth, he still needs a lot of closeness and cuddling to help him adjust to his new surroundings. Some people think that by holding babies too much you can spoil them. But tiny babies have only their parents to count on to take care of their needs, and they have only one way to communicate—by crying. When you respond to your baby's cry, he learns that someone is there for him and he is given a clear message that he is loved. Responding to your baby's needs builds his trust in people and makes him feel more secure. Studies show that babies who are held often cry fewer hours per day and are more self-confident as they mature.

6. Are my breasts too small (or large) to breastfeed?

Fortunately, making enough milk for your baby does not depend on the size of your breasts. The size of your breasts is determined by the amount of **fatty tissue** you have in your breasts. Breast milk is made by the **glandular tissue** in your breasts, *not* the fatty tissue. So size has nothing to do with the amount of milk you can make. Almost all women are born with enough glandular tissue to breastfeed. When you become pregnant, your body thinks you are going to breastfeed whether you do or not and your breasts prepare to make milk. After birth, hormonal changes in your body tell the glandular tissue in your breasts to produce milk. **Then it is the baby who controls how much milk you make—the more your baby nurses, the more milk you will have.**

7. Will breastfeeding change the shape and size of my breasts?

As soon as a woman becomes pregnant, permanent changes begin to occur in her breasts. What some mothers call "saggy" breasts are caused by an increase in breast size during pregnancy—and not caused by breastfeeding. Heredity, the elasticity of your skin, and the amount of weight you gain also affect how your breasts will look after pregnancy. Usually about 6 months after you have *weaned* (stopped breastfeeding), your breasts will return to more of their pre-pregnancy look. They will also feel firmer as fatty tissue begins to fill them out again. The great thing about breastfeeding is that you will finally meet someone who loves your breasts no matter how small, large, flat, flabby, or lopsided they are!

8. My mother didn't have enough milk—will I?

Many women feel they won't be able to make enough milk for their babies because their mothers weren't successful. But this really has nothing to do with *your* ability to breastfeed or make milk for *your* baby. Most likely, the reason your mother stopped breastfeeding was because she didn't have the correct information or the support she needed. You may feel pressure from mothers who formula-fed their children because they think you should too. But it is understandable that they may feel a little resentful because you are doing something they didn't do—and maybe wish they had. The times were most likely different when they were new mothers. If they had known all the things we know now about breastfeeding and had gotten help, they may have done things differently. Once you understand how breastfeeding works and you are convinced of the health benefits for you and your baby, stick to your decision and don't let friends or family members talk you out of it. Share the information you have learned with them and they will most likely support you. You will feel much more dedicated if you have at least one person you are close to who supports your decision to breastfeed, whether it's your partner, mother, sister, or a friend.

9. What if I don't make enough milk for my baby?

Most women can produce more than enough breast milk for their babies. Studies have shown that even malnourished women are able to make a sufficient amount of milk to nourish their growing infants. Most babies who gain weight slowly, or lose weight, are most likely not getting the milk their mothers are making. This is usually because the baby is not latched on to the breast correctly or is sucking improperly. In very rare cases—about 1 in 2,000—a mother doesn't have enough working glandular tissue to make enough milk to support her infant's growth. Also, some mothers who have had breast surgery may have had glandular tissue removed or affected in such a way that they cannot release the milk to their babies. But most mothers who "don't have enough milk" really don't have true physical problems such as these. Most likely, they are not getting the help they need and are giving their babies formula. When a baby receives formula instead of breast milk, it causes the mother's milk supply to slow down. If your milk supply is low because your baby wasn't getting your milk, this doesn't mean that you need to stop breastfeeding. See "Low Milk Supply" on PAGE 56 for help with increasing your milk supply. However, in some cases, you may need the help of a lactation specialist to get your milk flowing again.

10. Will my partner be jealous if I breastfeed?

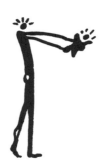

If you prepare your partner in advance about what to expect, he might be more open to the idea of breastfeeding. Let him know the important reasons you want to breastfeed and how it will benefit the whole family. Let him know how he won't have to get up in the middle of the night to help make bottles of formula and how much money your family will save—up to $150 a month, the cost of infant formula and bottle-feeding accessories. Explain how breastfeeding will give your baby the best possible start in life and that the benefits will last a lifetime. Sometimes fathers will become jealous because you are spending so much time with the baby. But whether you breastfeed or not, babies need a lot of attention! Invite your partner to sit with you while you nurse so that he will feel more involved. Let breastfeeding become family time. There are many other ways your partner can feel close to the baby besides feeding him. The baby's father can be the one who bathes the baby, takes him for a walk, and puts him to bed at night. He can burp, hold, and cuddle the baby, and change his diapers. Babies can never have too much love and attention from their fathers! Always remind your partner how important he is to both you and your baby. To give him a better idea of what to expect, have him read "What Can I Expect as a Breastfeeding Father?" on PAGE 14.

11. Will my partner find me less attractive if I breastfeed?

Some men may have trouble getting used to the idea of women's breasts being a source of nourishment as well as sexual stimulation. On the other hand, the idea of full breasts filled with "the milk of life" can be a very powerful thing. Many fathers enjoy watching the womanly way a mother nurses her child. Helping your partner understand that breastfeeding is a natural part of life will make it easier to gain his support. If your partner feels uncomfortable, it may help to talk to other breastfeeding couples so that he can become more familiar with these new images of breastfeeding and begin to understand that they are normal and healthy.

12. Will breastfeeding affect my sex life?

After the birth of a baby, most couples need time to get used to each other again sexually. For a while, lovemaking may be a little different from what you were used to before the baby. Much of this has to do with female hormones. Before having a baby, your *sexual hormones* are higher than your *mothering hormones*. After childbirth, and while you are breastfeeding, the opposite happens. Your mothering hormones kick in and your desire to take care of your baby may be stronger than your desire for sexual intimacy with your partner. This is quite normal and is nature's way of ensuring the survival of the species. But a woman's sexual responsiveness after childbirth varies from woman to woman. There may be times when your sexual desire is very high, and yet other times when you are too tired to even think about it. The important thing is to talk over your feelings with your partner and try to make time to be intimate. It may be difficult at first, but once your baby is a little older, your sexual hormones will kick in again and finding time to make love will become a lot easier. Mature parents realize that an infant has many needs—but those needs do lessen over time. The teamwork of caring for a newborn can actually bring a couple closer as they develop parenting skills together.

13. How long should I breastfeed my baby?

One of the best things you can do for your baby is to breastfeed as long as possible. The longer you breastfeed, the greater the benefits are for both you and your baby. **The American Academy of Pediatrics recommends breastfeeding for at least the first year of life.** They recommend feeding your baby only breast milk for the first 6 months, and then adding solid foods while continuing to breastfeed. The World Health Organization encourages mothers to breastfeed even longer than a year. Breastfed babies don't need any solid food or supplements of water, formula, juice, or other fluids for the first 6 months—just breast milk. No matter how old your baby is, each time he nurses, he will continue to receive *immunities* (disease fighting factors) and other benefits. So, *any* time you spend breastfeeding is better than none at all.

14. Do I have to drink a lot of milk to make milk for my baby?

A new mother does not need to drink milk to make milk for her baby. In fact, humans are the only species that drinks the milk of another species. When you think about it, the purpose of breast milk is to promote the best possible body growth and brain development of human infants, while the purpose of cow's milk is to promote the best possible body growth and brain development of baby calves. This could partly explain the lower obesity rates and higher IQs among breastfed children. Although drinking milk is not required, it is recommended that a nursing mother eat a balanced diet of grains, vegetables, fruits, protein, and calcium-rich foods. Calcium can be found in other dairy products besides milk, such as yogurt and cheese, or in nondairy foods such as turnip and mustard greens, fish with bones (salmon, sardines), broccoli, pinto beans, and corn tortillas. It can also be found in calcium-fortified cereals, tofu, and orange juice. In many countries, mothers don't drink milk at all and get all their calcium from these other sources.

15. Do I have to eat a special diet to breastfeed?

You do not have to eat a special diet in order to breastfeed. Even women in third-world countries whose diets include mostly rice successfully breastfeed. However, a breastfeeding mother should try to eat a balanced diet to keep up her energy and her own good health. Although no foods are off limits, a few mothers find that certain foods they eat seem to upset their babies (see "Foods that Can Sometimes Cause a Reaction" on PAGE 81). When food sensitivities do occur, it is usually in babies whose families have a history of allergies. The good news is that babies with food sensitivities usually outgrow them by 3 months of age. On the other hand, your baby may have no reaction to any foods at all. In fact, in many countries where spicy foods are commonly eaten, mothers breastfeed with no problems.

16. Will breastfeeding help me lose weight?

Most mothers find that they lose their pregnancy weight more quickly and easily while breastfeeding. This is because making breast milk burns a good number of calories—between 500 and 800 per day! Breastfeeding mothers can even eat a few more calories than non-breastfeeding mothers and still lose weight. Studies have shown that during the first 6 months after childbirth, breastfeeding mothers reach their pre-pregnancy weight sooner than their formula-feeding friends. The recommended rate of weight loss for breastfeeding mothers is 1 to 2 pounds per week. Obviously, there are healthy things you can do to help the weight come off, such as eat a balanced diet and exercise. See Chapter 6, "Nutrition for the Nursing Mother," to guide you on your way.

17. If I'm stressed, anxious, or not eating well, will it affect my milk?

Some mother's worry that if they are stressed or anxious, or if they eat poorly for a few days, it will affect their breast milk. But none of these things will affect your milk supply or the quality of your milk. Most women who tend to be tense or hyper can successfully breastfeed. In fact, the hormones your body makes during breastfeeding help you relax and feel calmer. Breastfeeding also calms your baby while he is nursing. So the quickest way to calm yourself and your baby is to put your baby to the breast. And malnutrition is rarely a cause of milk supply problems, because a mother's body has the amazing ability to protect and nourish her baby even when food is in short supply.

18. Can I smoke while breastfeeding?

Smoking is not a good habit no matter how you feed your baby. If you smoke, or your baby is around people who smoke, he will receive "second-hand" smoke. Second-hand smoke causes babies to have breathing problems and more coughs, colds, and ear infections. Also, babies who are around people who smoke have a higher risk of crib death (SIDS). The tobacco from cigarettes contain a drug called *nicotine* that passes into breast milk and may even affect the amount of milk the mother makes. Of course it would be better if you did not smoke, but if you cannot stop or cut down, it is better to breastfeed than to formula feed. Breastfeeding can keep babies who are around smoke from getting sick so often. If you do smoke, do it *after* you breastfeed, **not** *before*, and do not smoke near your baby. Breastfeeding is especially important for mothers who smoke because the benefits of breast milk still outweigh the risks from nicotine.

19. Can I drink alcohol while breastfeeding?

A mother can have some alcohol while breastfeeding. An occasional glass of wine or beer is not believed to harm a nursing infant—the key is moderation. Try to limit yourself to 1 or 2 drinks per week. Alcohol is a drug and passes through your breast milk to your baby and can cause him to be more wakeful and fussy if you overdo it. Having 2 or more drinks per day has been shown to cause delays in a baby's motor development. Also, studies have shown that having several drinks over a short period of time can immediately affect your baby's central nervous system and may affect your ability to produce milk. Besides, regular use of alcohol will affect your ability to care for your child. If you choose to drink, you can lessen the effects by nursing your baby just before you have a drink, and waiting at least 3 hours after drinking before nursing again. Remember, alcohol contains calories and has no nutritional value, so it's best to limit your alcohol use to special occasions.

20. Can I take medications or drugs while breastfeeding?

Most medications are safe to take while breastfeeding, but there are a few that can be dangerous for the baby when they pass through your breast milk. To be sure, let your doctor and your baby's doctor know that you are breastfeeding and get approval for all medications, including non-prescription drugs. Also, take the medication just after you nurse rather than just before. If your doctor says you must *wean* (stop breastfeeding) to take a certain drug, you may want to get a second opinion by contacting a lactation specialist for more information. Mood-altering drugs should not be taken by nursing mothers. Drugs such as marijuana, cocaine, PCP, heroin, and amphetamines can intoxicate the baby and he can become addicted to these drugs. These abusive drugs are dangerous and pose a very serious health risk to both the mother and the baby. Additionally, drug use and abuse seriously affects a mother's ability to care for her child.

21. Can I get pregnant while breastfeeding?

It is not a foolproof method, but breastfeeding can offer some protection from becoming pregnant, especially during the first 6 months after childbirth—if you are breastfeeding *exclusively* (giving your baby only breast milk) and you have not yet had a normal menstrual period. After the first 6 months, or once your menstrual cycle begins, the protection is less. When you breastfeed exclusively, your ovaries usually stop *ovulating* (releasing eggs) and your periods stop. This makes it harder for you to get pregnant. But there are no guarantees that you will not get pregnant while you are nursing, because sometimes you can ovulate without having a period first—making it possible to get pregnant. The only way to make sure you do not get pregnant is to use another method of birth control. If you choose the birth control pill, the safest one to use is the progesterone-only birth control pill called the "mini-pill." Talk to your doctor about which method of birth control is best for you.

22. Can I breastfeed while I'm pregnant?

You can still continue to breastfeed if you find out you are pregnant—unless you have a history of miscarriages or preterm labor with previous pregnancies. This is because breastfeeding causes the uterus to contract and may increase the risk of either one happening again. But studies have shown that in normal pregnancies there is no nutritional risk to the fetus or increased risk of miscarriage. So, you can nurse your child as long as you feel comfortable. However, some women decide to stop nursing when they become pregnant because their nipples become sensitive, or for other various reasons. But there is no medical reason you can't continue to breastfeed. Your milk supply may decrease during pregnancy, but if your baby is over 6 months old and already eating solid foods, this is usually not a problem.

23. Can I go back to work or school and still breastfeed?

If you plan to go back to work or school, breastfeeding is a perfect way to keep the strong connection you have with your baby while you are away. Even if you know you only have a few weeks to be home with your baby, give breastfeeding a try. Many new mothers who have to go back to work or school shortly after the delivery feel it is not worth it so they don't even try, or they give up just after a few days. But it is important to realize that these early days are the most critical days in your baby's life. Breastfeeding for just a few days or weeks is so much better than not breastfeeding at all. The health benefits for your baby are really worth it. You can learn to pump and express your breast milk so a caregiver can feed your baby your milk while you are away. Or if you choose, you can combine breastfeeding with formula feeding. See Chapter 8, "Working and Breastfeeding," beginning on PAGE 93 for more ideas on how to make it work.

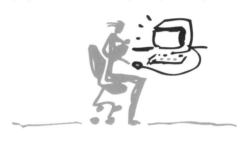

Why Is Breastfeeding So Important?

Understanding why good health begins with breastfeeding will help strengthen your commitment to nurse your baby. The more you know, the more likely you are to get off to a good start, and your baby can begin to enjoy the many health benefits and convenience of breastfeeding. The following section will explain why breastfeeding is so important, and it will also give you all the ammunition you need if you happen to run into someone who is questioning your decision to breastfeed.

There is clearly a difference between human breast milk and infant formula. Your breast milk was designed to provide your baby with the best possible nutrition for proper growth and brain development. Breast milk also contains live immune factors called *antibodies*. **Antibodies** are special proteins that help protect your baby from infections and diseases until his own immune system is fully developed. Infant formulas do not offer this protection because live antibodies can *never* be duplicated in infant formulas. Because of the protection received from these antibodies, breastfed children have less of the following:

- colds and viruses
- vomiting
- spitting up
- diarrhea
- constipation
- allergies
- diaper rash
- eczema
- asthma
- ear infections
- respiratory tract infections
- gastrointestinal infections

Studies have also shown that breastfed children have reduced risk of:

- crib death (SIDS)
- childhood cancers
- diabetes
- obesity

Besides this, your baby is able to digest the proteins in breast milk more quickly, easily, and efficiently than the proteins found in infant formulas. Studies have also found that children who are breastfed have higher IQs than formula-fed children. Additionally, the special sucking at the breast provides good jaw and tooth development.

Some women think that when they are sick, they should not breastfeed their babies. But most common illnesses, such as a cold or the flu, cannot be passed from the mother to the baby through breast milk. In fact, if you are sick, your breast milk will protect your baby from getting the same illness. When a mother becomes ill, her body produces special antibodies to fight that specific illness. These antibodies pass through her breast milk to protect her baby from the same illness.

There are also many health benefits for you, the nursing mother. The longer you breastfeed your baby, the less risk you have of the following:

- pre-menopausal breast cancer
- ovarian cancer
- cervical cancer
- osteoporosis (weakening of the bones)

Additionally, breastfeeding helps with your recovery after childbirth. While you are breastfeeding, your uterus shrinks back to its pre-pregnancy size more quickly and there is less blood loss. Breastfeeding also burns calories, so it can help you get back to your pre-pregnancy weight more quickly. The return of your period is also delayed while you are breastfeeding, which may help lengthen the time between pregnancies.

Remember that breastfeeding is much more than just nourishment. Nursing is a way of developing a special relationship with your baby and gives him much comfort and security. When you and your baby form a loving circle of skin-to-skin contact, it helps reduce the stress he feels after leaving the security of your womb to enter his new world.

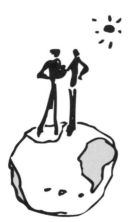

And a breastfed baby always knows who his mother is. Even if you have to go back to work or school, you don't have to worry that he will become too attached to his caregiver. Breastfeeding as often as you can when you are together will help you keep a strong emotional connection to your baby.

There are also many practical reasons to nurse your baby. Breastfeeding is convenient, saves time, money, and energy. It is always instantly available, fresh, sterile, and at the right temperature—which makes going out with your baby especially easy. It is friendlier to the environment because it saves energy and does not produce packaging waste. Breastfeeding also cuts down on national health care costs, contributes to a more productive workforce, and creates a stronger and healthier society.

Overall, your breastfed baby will be healthier—and a healthy baby is a happy baby! As a result, you will have fewer medical bills, fewer missed days of work, and fewer nights of interrupted sleep because of a sick infant. By breastfeeding, you are giving your baby a strong foundation for a lifetime of good health, while creating a strong emotional bond. No one loves your baby like you, and breastfeeding is a once-in-a-lifetime experience that only you can give your baby.

What Can I Expect as a Breastfeeding Mother?

Whether or not you choose to breastfeed, caring for a new baby is probably the most difficult job you will ever have. But along with it come many rewards and joys. Being a new mother is very exciting, but at times, it can also be very overwhelming and exhausting. Taking care of yourself is very important. Realize that during the first 6 weeks after the delivery you will be recovering from pregnancy and childbirth—both physically and emotionally. Try to eat well, rest when you can, and take one day at a time.

As you get used to your new role as mother, help from your partner will be very important, especially during the early days. Some fathers aren't sure how they feel about breastfeeding because of the mixed messages we have in our society about sexuality and breastfeeding. Your partner may enjoy watching you nurse and bond with your baby, or he may feel uncomfortable and threatened by how close the two of you are. He may come to like the idea of breastfeeding once he knows all the benefits, yet he still may be uneasy when you need to nurse around other people.

If your partner is feeling uncomfortable, the best thing to do is explain to him why breastfeeding is so important to you and get him involved with the baby from the very beginning. During the early weeks you may find that your bond with your baby is so strong that you don't want to share baby care with any one else. But it is important to step back and let your partner develop his own relationship with the baby. Too many fathers feel left out from day one and have a hard time jumping back in.

Give your partner every chance to hold, comfort, bathe, dress, burp, entertain, and change the baby—if he is willing. This will help him build his own confidence in caring for his child, and you will know the baby is in good hands while you take a shower or nap. Just realize that your partner's parenting style may be different from yours. You may want to look over his shoulder and be critical, but unless he asks for your help, let him do things his own way so he can develop his own parenting skills. If his parenting skills aren't bothering the baby, hopefully, they won't bother you. Remember, his relationship with your child from infancy has an important affect on your child's growth and development. Your child's early emotional attachment to his father will help to build a strong family bond.

Make sure you let your partner know that you appreciate his help and support. Tell him how lucky your child is to have him as a father. Thank him for helping around the house, and for understanding that this demanding newborn period won't last forever. Assure him that you will be able to breastfeed discreetly so that no one becomes uncomfortable. Let him know how important he is to the success of your breastfeeding relationship.

For some new mothers, getting their partners involved with the baby may not be so easy. There are some fathers who are just not comfortable handling a newborn and are not ready to jump right in and help out with baby care. Holding and comforting the baby may be all that he is able to do at first. But don't worry, he will have many more chances to become comfortable handling the baby as the baby grows and becomes more responsive. He can still be a big help by doing household chores. If you feel that you will need more help than your partner is able to give during the early weeks, arrange to have a friend or family member stay with you after your baby is born.

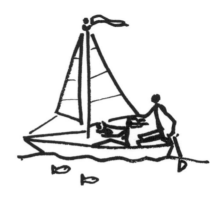

Just remember that all new mothers need help. Whether it's having a friend listen to your childbirth story or a relative help you clean your house—you need to reach out to other people. You need to feel connected to the outside world. You need to express your feelings and be heard. You need to share your experiences and compare notes with other mothers. You need reassurance that you are doing things right. But most of all, in order to make it through these early weeks, you need loving care from those around you. Creating this circle of support will make nursing your baby a more positive experience. The rewards of all your work will come once you are through the rough waters of the hectic first few weeks. There will be smooth sailing ahead on your way to becoming a happy breastfeeding family.

What Can I Expect as a Breastfeeding Father?

Many fathers think that breastfeeding doesn't have anything to do with them, since they are not actually feeding the baby. But as the baby's father, you play a very important role in your partner's breastfeeding success. Your encouragement and support will help your partner feel better about herself and be proud that she is giving your baby the very best. Breastfeeding is a natural part of life and the most fatherly thing you can do is to support your partner in her new role as a breastfeeding mother. Try to arrange to take off as much time as possible to be with your new family during the early weeks. Help her with household chores so that she can give her full attention to learning how to nurse your baby. Make sure your partner eats well and rests, and help her with baby care responsibilities. Take every chance to hold, comfort, bathe, dress, burp, entertain, and change your baby—this is your chance to start developing your own special relationship. Caring for your baby during these early years will have a positive influence on his future growth and development and will create a strong family bond.

Understand that breastfeeding is physically and emotionally demanding and that your partner will be spending most of her time with the baby. It is completely normal to feel left out at times and wonder if you will ever have your partner back. You may also worry that you won't be able to develop your own relationship with your baby. Some men feel so uncomfortable with breastfeeding that they encourage bottle feeding. But education is the key. Hopefully, once you see the advantages of breastfeeding for your entire family, you will want to do what ever it takes to help your partner be successful. Learn as much as you can about breastfeeding. Read this book and attend prenatal and breastfeeding classes with your partner. Once you are convinced that "breast is best" for your baby, it will be easier for you to be supportive.

Remember that your partner is recovering from the physical demands of pregnancy and childbirth and adjusting to hormonal changes in her body. These hormonal changes may affect her mood. She may be more irritable, forgetful, and distracted, and she may be less interested in sex. Expect that it will take a little time to start up your sexual relationship again. Share your feelings with your partner and plan time to be intimate. Before long, her hormones will shift back, your baby will be less demanding, and you will have your partner back. Your relationship may even be stronger than before—especially if you've been sensitive and supportive!

As a new father, a lot of demands are being put upon you and at times it may seem difficult and overwhelming. Look to friends and family members for emotional support and reassurance. It helps to talk to other breastfeeding fathers so you can share your feelings. Once you accept your new role as a father, you will find yourself rising to the occasion and feeling proud of the valuable contribution you are making to your new family. Later on down the road, as you look at your growing child, you will be glad you supported breastfeeding.

Finally, appreciate the advantages of having a breastfed baby. Your child will be healthier and you will have fewer medical expenses. Your nights will be less interrupted, since you won't have to get up for middle-of-the-night bottle feedings. Outings will be much easier for everyone. And just think of all the money you will save—because breastfeeding is free!

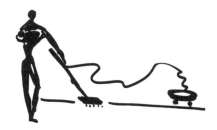

CHAPTER 2

Breastfeeding Basics

Preparing For Breastfeeding

You may be wondering why there is so much more to learn about breastfeeding than formula feeding. The answer is that even though breastfeeding is natural, it doesn't always come naturally to mothers or babies. In our culture we are not used to seeing mothers nurse their infants openly, so most new mothers need help figuring it out. Also, unlike a bottle, breast milk doesn't just drip out of our breasts. Our babies need to learn how to take the milk from our breasts, and we need to learn how to help them along. Just know that it may take a little while for both you and your new baby to figure out what to do. Taking the time to learn all you can *before* your baby arrives can make breastfeeding go more smoothly for both of you.

Talk to Your Doctor

Talk to your doctor about breastfeeding before your baby arrives. If you decide to breastfeed, your doctor can examine your breasts and nipples to reassure you that you are able to nurse your baby. If you have had any type of breast surgery, you may need extra help. In some cases, the *glandular tissue* (where the milk is made) is affected during surgery, so it is important to work closely with your doctor or a lactation specialist after the delivery to make sure your baby is getting enough breast milk.

Check Your Nipple Type

There is great variation in women's nipples. It is helpful to know if your nipples are *normal*, *flat*, or *inverted*. Some women have nipples that *invert* (go in) when they are pinched. This makes it harder for the baby to latch on to the breast and take it into his mouth. To find out if you have inverted nipples, gently pinch the base of your nipple. An **inverted nipple** will go in when it is pinched, while a **normal nipple** will stick out. A **flat nipple** looks flat but sticks out slightly.

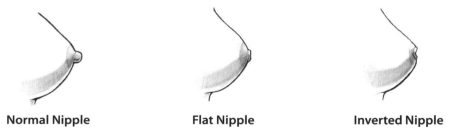

Normal Nipple   **Flat Nipple**   **Inverted Nipple**

The problem of inverted nipples usually clears up on its own during pregnancy as your breasts get larger. If it doesn't clear up, you may still be able to gently pull your nipples out with your fingers (just far enough for the baby to latch on to) before you nurse.

If you think you may have difficulty with inverted nipples, or you have flat nipples, seek the advice of your doctor or a lactation specialist who may recommend the use of *breast shells*. **Breast shells** are round plastic shells that fit over your breasts and can be worn in your bra during the last months of pregnancy and between feedings to help bring out your nipples. They work by putting pressure around the base of the nipple, which pushes the nipple outward. *Nipple shields* can also help a baby who is having problems grasping the mother's nipple. **Nipple shields** are made of soft silicon and can be worn over a mother's nipple during feedings. However, nipple shields should only be used under the guidance of a lactation specialist or someone who is knowledgeable about special breastfeeding situations.

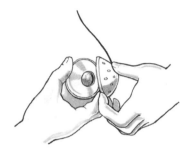

Breast Shell

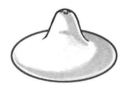

Nipple Shield

Prepare Your Breasts

There is very little you need to do to prepare your breasts for breastfeeding. During pregnancy, just make sure your bras provide enough support. There is no need to toughen your nipples or *express* (take milk out of) your breasts prior to delivery. These things can, in fact, bring on labor. Just wash your breasts with plain warm water. Soaps, lotions, and alcohol are not necessary. Your nipples are already making what they need for their protection. The small bumps on your areola called the *Montgomery glands* produce a special oil that naturally cleans, lubricates, and protects the nipple. Wash your hands before each feeding, and if you wear nursing pads, change them often. If your nipples feel chapped, dry, or itchy, you can use 100% modified lanolin for nursing mothers available at most major drug stores. It soothes, moisturizes, and heals sore nipples by helping the skin keep its inner moisture.

Learn as Much as You Can

Educate yourself about breastfeeding *before* your baby arrives. Read books and pamphlets, watch videos, and talk to other women who have breastfed. Take a breastfeeding class if you can and have your partner or other support person attend the class with you. Try to attend a La Leche League meeting while you are still pregnant. La Leche League International is a worldwide organization that helps families learn about breastfeeding. The meet-

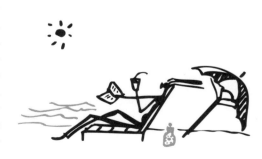

ings are held once a month and are open to the public. At a meeting you will meet other mothers who are breastfeeding. You will be able to watch them nurse their babies and talk to them about breastfeeding. You will also have someone to call on if you have questions or need help after your baby is born.

Set Up a Support System

Realize that you will need some help for several days, or even weeks, after giving birth. Arrange for family and friends to help with household chores, meals, and running errands so that you can spend your time and energy caring for your newborn. Also, knowing where to turn for breastfeeding help if you have problems will be very important. The following are people and organizations that help breastfeeding mothers:

- Your doctor
- Your baby's doctor
- Your local health department
- Your local WIC clinic
- A lactation specialist which may include:
  - a La Leche League Leader or Peer Counselor
  - a WIC Breastfeeding Counselor or Peer Counselor
  - an International Board Certified Lactation Consultant (IBCLC)
  - other certified lactation specialist

How Breastfeeding Works

By understanding how breastfeeding works, you will know what to expect during the early days. It will also make it easier to solve any problems you may have. How your body makes milk for your baby is based on the principle of *supply and demand*. What this means is that after your baby takes the milk from your breasts, **the demand**, it is automatically replaced by a fresh batch, **the supply**. The amount of milk your baby takes from your breasts and how often your baby nurses is what tells your body how much milk to make. **The more often your baby nurses and the more milk he takes, the more milk your body will make.**

During the early weeks of nursing, it is important not to give your baby anything other than milk from your breasts. Giving your baby bottles of formula or water, will throw off the delicate balance of supply and demand. If you fill up your baby's tummy with formula or water, he will want less breast milk from you. Then, because the demand on your body is lowered, you will make less milk. This in turn will cause you to give him even more formula or water. As you can see, if you continue this cycle, your milk supply will slow down and eventually stop, causing an early end to breastfeeding. **Breastfeeding often—***and only breastfeeding***—is what creates a good milk supply.**

It is also advised not to offer your baby a bottle or pacifier until he is 3 to 4 weeks old, or at least until you have a good milk supply and your baby is latching on well. Artificial nipples require a different sucking pattern than breastfeeding and the baby may become confused about how to suck at the breast. In the early weeks, all of your baby's sucking should be done at the breast. Remember breastfeeding often and only breastfeeding is what creates a good milk supply. If your baby is not able to nurse at the breast, it is best to feed him your pumped breast milk with a spoon, small cup, medicine dropper, or nursing supplementer, until he is at least 3 to 4 weeks old.

How Your Breasts Make Milk

Humans are known as **mammals** because we have **mammary glands** (also known as breasts) to make milk for our young. When you become pregnant, your breasts become tender as they naturally start preparing to make milk for your baby. Toward the middle of your pregnancy, your breasts become larger, the areolas darker, and the veins under the skin more visible. The *Montgomery glands* on your areolas also become active and start producing an oily-like substance that helps keep the skin around your nipples soft and discourages the growth of bacteria. Toward the end of your pregnancy, your breasts start producing *colostrum*—a thick, yellow fluid that provides your baby with his first feedings.

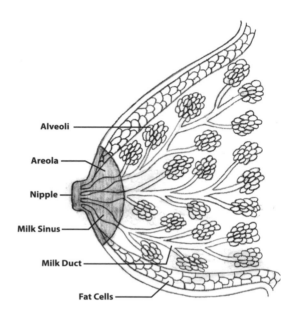

The *glandular tissue* in your breasts is where the milk is made. The **glandular tissue** is made up of *alveoli, milk ducts,* and *milk sinuses*. The milk is made in the **alveoli** (grape-like clusters of cells), and then travels down the **milk ducts** to the **milk sinuses** where it stays until you nurse your baby. The milk sinuses are found beneath the areola. The milk empties from the sinuses through about 15 to 20 openings in your nipple and into your baby's mouth. To empty the milk sinuses, your baby's gums must be positioned over the areola so that his jaws press on these sinuses where the milk is stored. For this reason, your baby should have the nipple and at least 1 to 1½ inches of your areola in his mouth—not *just* the nipple. If your baby sucks only on the nipple, very little milk will come out and your nipple will become sore.

The Let-down (or Milk-ejection) Reflex

When your baby sucks at your breast, the nerves inside your nipple send a message to your brain. When your brain receives this message, it tells the pituitary gland to release two hormones: *prolactin* and *oxytocin*. **Prolactin** causes the alveoli in your breasts to make milk. **Oxytocin** causes the muscle fibers around the alveoli to contract, which sends the milk down through the milk ducts into the milk sinuses under the areola tissue. As your baby sucks your breast and presses on the milk sinuses, the milk is released through the openings in your nipple and into the back of your baby's mouth. This sudden release of milk is called the let-down or milk-ejection reflex.

Arriving at the Hospital

Breastfeeding right after birth helps to ensure that you get off to the right start. When you arrive at the hospital, make sure the nursing staff knows that you want to breastfeed your baby immediately after birth. Let them know that you don't want your baby to have any bottles of formula, sugar water, or pacifiers while in the hospital. A baby who is given an artificial nipple in the hospital may have trouble learning how to breastfeed, since breastfeeding requires more work than sucking on an artificial nipple.

To make it easier for you, your partner can attach the **"Breastfeeding Baby in Training"** sign (on PAGE 23) to your baby's bassinet while you are in the hospital. This will make your wish to nurse your baby very clear to the hospital staff. The nursing staff can change many times during your hospital stay and you may be too exhausted to repeat yourself. The rewards of breastfeeding are far too valuable to get off to the wrong start because you weren't able to express your needs. **Even though you may not spend much time in the hospital, the first 2 to 3 days after the delivery are the most important days in getting off to the right start with breastfeeding.**

Rooming-in

Find out if your hospital has *rooming-in*. **Rooming-in** is when new mothers are able to have their babies in their rooms with them for all or most of their hospital stay. This allows you and your baby to get more practice breastfeeding and will give you a chance to get in tune with each other early on. If your hospital doesn't have rooming-in, you can tell the nurses that you would like to keep your baby in your room with you most of the time. Or you can have them bring your baby to you often, especially when he wants to nurse. Most problems that happen because of hospital routines, such as nurses giving babies bottles or pacifiers, can be prevented if your baby is able to stay with you.

A Baby Is Born

After nine long months, the moment you have all been waiting for has finally arrived—your baby has made his grand entrance into the world! You have just been through one of the most difficult yet amazing experiences of your life. You have given birth to a beautiful new human being. Now the real work—and the joy—begin. By giving your baby your loving attention during these early years, you will plant the seeds for him to grow and become a confident, secure, and loving person. As you help your child become a person, he will help you become a parent. Now it is time to introduce yourself to your baby and start the mothering process.

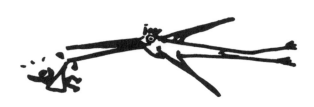

Your Baby's First Feeding

Right after birth, babies are in a quiet, alert state and most babies are ready and willing to nurse. After the first hour, they become sleepy and it's harder to get them to nurse. Breastfeeding immediately after birth allows a baby to *imprint* on his mother's nipple, which has been shown to increase breastfeeding success. **Imprinting** is when a baby's first impressions of his mother have a lasting effect. When he nurses during this early alert period, he quickly learns what to do and who his mother is. Also during this time, his natural sucking reflex is strongest. Some babies may just nuzzle and lick the nipple instead of latching on. If this happens, don't worry, the closeness and warmth of the skin-to-skin contact will be comforting to your baby. You can try again in a half-hour or so. Remember, breastfeeding is a learning process for both of you—it may take a few times before your baby latches on well.

Colostrum

The first milk your body makes is called *colostrum*. **Colostrum** is thick and yellow and made in small amounts. It is high in protein and low in fat and contains a high concentration of antibodies. Your baby is born with extra fat and fluids in his body to help nourish him during the first 2 to 3 days of life, so small, frequent meals of colostrum is all he needs. Nursing often during the first few days will help bring in a good milk supply by the third or fourth day when colostrum begins to change into mature milk. Colostrum is a natural laxative and helps clean out your baby's intestines of **meconium**, your baby's first stools (poops). Colostrum also helps to get rid of the build up of **bilirubin**, the cause of *jaundice* (see "Jaundice" on PAGE 46). Colostrum is sometimes called "liquid gold" and may be considered your child's first immunization because of its many antibodies that protect your baby from diseases and infections.

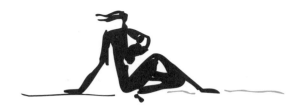

Breastfeeding Baby in Training

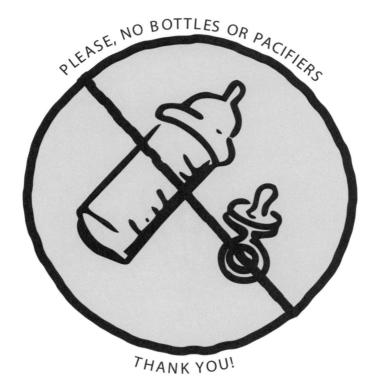

PLEASE, NO BOTTLES OR PACIFIERS

THANK YOU!

Baby's Name _____

Mother's Name _____

Room # _____

Bon Appétit, Baby!

Copyright © 2005 by Elaine Moran

Attach this sign to your baby's bassinet while in the hospital.

Latch-on

Getting your baby to latch on correctly is one of the most important ways to be successful at breastfeeding. Once you have learned how to position your baby, and your baby has learned how to latch on correctly, you are on your way! Just remember that some babies take longer than others to learn how to latch on and coordinate sucking, swallowing, and breathing. You just have to keep trying until your baby gets the hang of it. Before you know it, he will be a breastfeeding pro. Just make sure that you are relaxed and comfortable and that your baby is in the mood for nursing. If he is crying or upset, calm him down and comfort him before trying again.

To start a feeding, get into a comfortable breastfeeding position (see "Breastfeeding Positions" on PAGES 26–28), then follow these steps:

- Express a little colostrum from your breast onto your nipple.
- Hold your breast using your thumb and four fingers in the form of the letter "C" or "U" about 1 to 1½ inches back from the nipple.
- Gently squeeze and shape the breast so that it will fit easily into your baby's open mouth.
- Tickle the center of your baby's lips with your nipple until he opens his mouth wide, as in a yawn.
- When your baby opens wide and drops his lower jaw, quickly pull him in toward you and onto your breast, lower jaw first, so that he takes as much of your nipple and areola into his mouth as possible.
- Make sure you pull your baby in toward you. Leaning toward your baby may cause neck and back strain and incorrect latch-on.

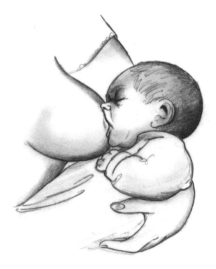

Correct Latch-on

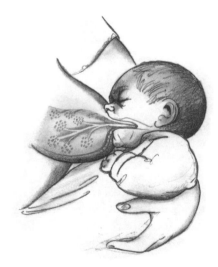

Inside View

Your baby is latched on well if both his lips are curved outward over your breast creating a good seal, and he has 1 to 1½ inches of your breast tissue in his mouth. As you can see from the "Inside View" above, when your baby opens wide and takes in your nipple and breast, he stretches the breast tissue so the nipple is far back in his mouth and does not rub on his tongue or gums. The tip of his nose and chin should be gently touching your breast. His lower jaw will do most of the work getting the milk from your breast. When he moves his lower jaw, it presses on the milk sinuses under your areola sending milk out through the tiny holes in your nipple and into the back of your baby's mouth. You should feel comfortable as your baby takes long drawing sucks and can be heard swallowing. You should **not** hear smacking, clicking, or slurping sounds. If your baby's sucking is painful, the position is not correct. Release your baby from your breast by gently putting your finger into the corner of his mouth to break the suction, and try again.

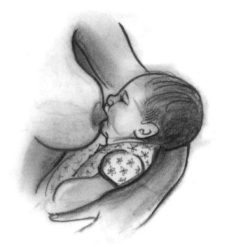

Incorrect Latch-on

Your baby is **not** latched on correctly if he is not taking enough of the areola into his mouth and is sucking only on the nipple. If this happens, your baby's tongue and gums will rub the sensitive skin of your nipple each time he sucks and you will end up with sore nipples. Also, your baby will have a hard time getting enough milk from your breasts to grow properly.

Once your baby is latched on correctly, let him nurse until he gets sleepy or pulls off on his own, then offer him the other breast. During these first nursing sessions, he may suck for only a few minutes at each breast or nurse only on one breast. This is normal. If you are having problems getting your baby to latch on, ask for help from a nurse or lactation specialist. By watching you breastfeed, she can tell you where the problem is and help you correct it early on. **While in the hospital your baby should be given a general health check-up and breastfeeding evaluation during the first 24 to 48 hours after birth.** Ask all the questions you can while you are in the hospital so that you can build your confidence before going home with your baby. Also, ask the hospital staff who you can call if you have questions or problems when you get home.

Breastfeeding Positions

Once you get the hang of it, getting your baby started at the breast will become very natural and easy. It takes much longer to describe the process than it actually does to do it. The most important thing is to get the baby positioned correctly from the start.

The following are descriptions of some of the most basic breastfeeding positions. During the early days of nursing, one position may be more comfortable for you than another. Later on, you might find that other positions work better in different situations. You don't have to use the same position every time you nurse. It is best to try each one to see what works best for you and your baby.

Cradle Hold. In this position you hold your baby's head in the bend of your elbow and "cradle" the infant. This classic breastfeeding position is the one most experienced nursing mothers find the easiest to use. Here are some tips for good positioning in the cradle hold.

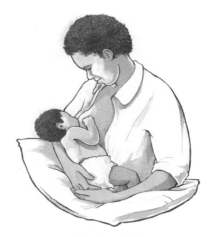

Cradle Hold

- Sit upright in a comfortable position. Place one or two pillows on your lap to bring your baby level with your nipple and to support your baby's weight. You can also put pillows behind your back for extra support.
- Cradle your baby with his head in the bend of your elbow.
- Turn your baby on his side so that his whole body is facing you and you are tummy-to-tummy. His knees should be pulled in close to your body and his lower arm can be placed around your waist.
- Support his back with your forearm and cup his buttocks or thigh with your hand. His body should be in a straight line. He should not have to turn his head sideways to reach your breast. This makes it very difficult to swallow (try swallowing while turning your head and you will see how difficult it is).
- When your baby opens his mouth wide, pull your baby in toward you and onto your breast so that he can latch on.

Cross Cradle Hold. (Also known as the *crossover* or *transition hold*.) During the early days of nursing, the cross cradle hold may be a more comfortable position for some new mothers. This position makes it easier for the mother to guide the baby's head to the breast with her hand, when his muscles aren't quite developed enough for him to latch on without help. In the cross cradle hold position you use the arm opposite the breast you are offering to support the length of the baby's back. His buttocks are at the bend of your elbow and the back of his head and neck rest on your hand. Here are some tips for good positioning in the cross cradle hold:

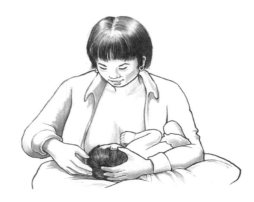

Cross Cradle Hold

- Sit upright in a comfortable position. Place one or two pillows on your lap to bring your baby level with your nipple and to support your baby's weight. You can also put pillows behind your back for extra support.
- Support your baby's body with the arm opposite the breast you are offering. The palm of your hand should be positioned between his shoulder blades, while supporting the back of his head and neck.

- Position your baby on his side so that his chest and tummy are against your body and his nose is facing your breast.
- When your baby opens his mouth wide, pull your baby in toward you and onto your breast so that he can latch on.

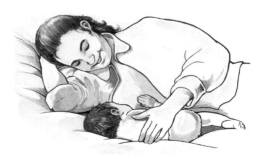

Side-lying Position

Side-lying Position. This position is recommended after a cesarean delivery, since it helps keep pressure off the abdomen. It is also great for nighttime nursing and a good way to get some rest during the day. In this position you and your baby are lying side-by-side facing each other. The baby is pulled in close, with his head at nipple level. Use pillows between your knees and along your back for extra support. Support your baby's back with your arm or place a rolled-up blanket behind his back.

Football Hold (also known as the *clutch hold*). Like the cross cradle hold, this position gives you better control of your baby's head and may be easier for you during the early days of nursing or after a cesarean delivery. In the football hold position, you are sitting upright and your baby is tucked under your arm like a football. Your baby's legs are behind you, and his face is looking up at you. Use pillows under your arm and under your baby so that he is at nipple level. You can also put pillows behind your back for extra support. Support your baby's head with your hand and use the opposite hand to support your breast.

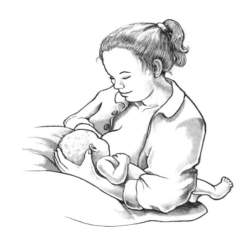

Football Hold

How Often Should I Nurse While in the Hospital?

While you are in the hospital, breastfeed your baby every 1½ to 3 hours, or at least 10 to 12 times every 24 hours. Let him nurse for as long as he wants. During the first day or two, while your baby receives colostrum, it is normal for him to nurse for only a short time at each breast (5 to 10 minutes), although some babies may nurse longer. Nursing often during the first couple of days will ensure that your baby gets the rich colostrum that is so important for his good health, and it will lessen his chances of getting jaundice. Frequent nursing also stimulates your breasts to begin making **mature milk,** which usually comes in about 2 to 3 days after giving birth. Also, early problems with engorgement and painful breasts may be prevented by nursing frequently. Offer both breasts at each feeding so that they are evenly stimulated to produce milk. However, it is fine if your baby takes only one breast. After each feeding, note which breast your baby took the *least* milk from and offer that breast *first* at next feeding.

Feeding times are measured from the *beginning* of one feeding session to the *beginning* of the next. For example, if your baby nursed from 1:00 p.m. to 1:15 p.m., and then again from 3:30 p.m. to 3:50 p.m., the time between these two feedings is 2½ hours—the time between the beginning of the first feeding session (1:00 p.m.) to the beginning of the next (3:30 p.m.).

These first days of nursing will give both you and your baby the time to get to know each other and practice working together as a team before your mature milk comes in. You will have a chance to practice good positioning and your baby will learn how to latch on correctly while your nipples are still soft and easy to grasp. These early days of nursing are your on-the-job-training for the task ahead. This beginning period seems to be Mother Nature's way of easing you both into the nursing relationship.

Signs of Hunger

Newborns count on their mothers to read their hunger signs. Your baby may show signs of hunger up to 30 minutes before he actually begins to cry. **These hunger signs may include fussing, sucking on his fingers or fist, brushing his hand across his face, making little sucking motions, or *rooting***—turning his head and opening his mouth as if he is searching for the nipple. It is important to read his hunger signs before he becomes too frustrated and upset to latch on properly. If you happen to miss these signs, you will soon hear his hunger cry—his only other way to communicate. Responding to your baby will allow him to develop a sense of trust in others. Knowing that he can influence his world will help him begin to build his own self-confidence. Even if at times you are unable to soothe your baby, continuing to try to comfort him will give him a sense that people care about how he feels and are there for him.

Burping

Breastfed babies don't swallow much air while nursing and some babies may not burp at all during or after a feeding. However, sometimes your newborn may gulp down his meal and swallow too much air, which can make him feel uncomfortably full before he has finished eating. After your baby has finished nursing on one breast, try burping him before offering the other. Burping your baby requires placing firm pressure on his tummy. The basic burping position is to hold your baby firmly against your shoulder while supporting his buttocks with one hand and patting or rubbing his back with the other. If your baby does not burp in a minute or two and he seems comfortable, there is no need for concern, just continue with the feeding.

Hiccups

All babies have hiccups from time to time, and some babies may hiccup more than others. Babies even hiccup inside the womb. But unlike adult hiccups, there is no known cause for newborn hiccups. But as annoying as they may seem to us, they are not bothersome for your baby. Breastfeeding will usually settle the spell, or the hiccups will eventually stop on their own.

Waking the Sleepy Baby

After the initial period of alertness during the first hour after birth, newborns often become very sleepy for the next several days. Some babies would rather sleep than nurse.

These sleepy babies do not eat as often as they should to grow properly, and when they do nurse, they may take only a few sucks before going right back to sleep. **It is important for mothers to wake a sleepy baby for feedings during the first 4 weeks. If your baby sleeps longer than 4 hours, it is necessary to wake him for a feeding.** It is easiest to wake your baby when he is in a light sleep cycle. Watch for eye movements under the eyelids, sucking movements, or restlessness. Then gently wake your baby by changing his diaper, rubbing his back, or massaging his feet while softly talking to him. If your baby falls asleep after only a few sucks at the breast, try *switch nursing*—as soon as your baby begins to lose interest in sucking, take him off the breast, burp him, and then latch him on to the other side. Repeat this 2 or 3 times during the feeding. With a sleepy baby the mother needs to take the lead and make sure her newborn nurses often enough. **The best way to tell if a sleepy baby is getting enough nourishment from breast milk is to check the amount of weight gain and number of wet and soiled (dirty) diapers.** (See "Is Your Baby Getting Enough?" on PAGE 35.)

Meconium

Meconium is the greenish-black, sticky, tar-like substance that fills your baby's intestines while he is in the womb. The colostrum that your baby is receiving acts as a laxative and helps clean out the meconium, your baby's first stools (poops). **Your newborn should have at least 1 meconium stool on Day 1 (the first 24 hours after birth).** He will continue to pass small amounts of meconium over the next 2 to 3 days. This is a good sign that he is getting enough colostrum and his digestive system is working properly. Call your baby's doctor if none has passed by Day 2.

Wet Diapers

Even if your baby started breastfeeding during the first hour after birth and is nursing often and well, it is normal for your baby not to have many wet diapers for the first 2 to 3 days. **However, your baby should have at least 1 to 2 wet diapers on Day 1 (the first 24 hours after birth.** On Day 2, again, he should have at least 1 to 2 wet diapers. Then by Day 3, his wet diapers should start to increase. This will ensure that he is getting enough colostrum. His urine (pee) should be pale yellow to almost clear in color.

Weight Gain

In the first 3 to 4 days after birth, it is normal for babies to lose about 7 percent of their birth weight. Babies are born with extra fluid, which they quickly lose during the first few days of life. Once your mature milk comes in, and your milk supply increases, expect your baby to start gaining weight. **After the initial weight loss, your baby should be back up to his birth weight by about 2 weeks of age. Then he should gain approximately 4 to 7 ounces per week, or at least one pound per month.** This is one of the best ways to tell if your baby is getting enough breast milk. Be sure to count weight gain from his lowest weight (his weight on the third or fourth day of life), not from his birth weight. Watching your baby's growth pattern is another way of checking his overall health. But keep in mind that the rate and steadiness of growth is more important than the actual amount of growth.

At Home With Your Baby

Once you are home from the hospital, plan to spend much of your time comforting and nursing your newborn. The first 6 weeks *postpartum* (after the baby's birth) is the time for developing a healthy nursing relationship. You will probably notice that your newborn's life consists of little more than nursing, sleeping, waking, crying, and eliminating (peeing and pooping). This is your baby's job for these first few weeks—and your job is to make sure he is growing and developing. **It is recommended that a breastfed baby have a follow-up visit by a health care professional (a doctor, nurse, or lactation specialist) at 2 to 4 days of age to be weighed and to make sure everything is going well.** If you are not sure your baby is breastfeeding well, the health care professional can watch a feeding so that any problems can be corrected immediately. **By 5 to 7 days of age, it is recommended that your baby be seen by a doctor to be weighed and checked for jaundice and to make sure he is having enough wet and soiled diapers.**

While at home, it is important that your baby's surroundings are as calm and comfortable as possible. Your newborn has just arrived from an amazing journey. He has gone through a big change from the comfort of your womb, to the bright lights of the hospital, to the journey home. He is trying to get used to his strange new world. He is now required to breathe and digest on his own, while adjusting to the new sensations of touch, light, odors, and unfamiliar sounds. Keeping your newborn's surroundings as calm and quiet as possible for the first several days will prevent over-stimulation and gently ease him into life outside the womb.

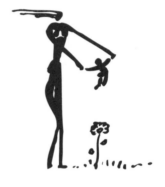

It is natural for new parents to feel a little uneasy about caring for their newborns once they are at home. A new baby doesn't come with an instruction manual, and people often become parents without any previous experience with babies. But with a little time and practice, you will overcome the insecurity that comes with being a new parent—experience is the best teacher. When parents are calm and secure it rubs off on the baby.

Just remember that all babies are different and have their own unique personalities. You can read as much as you can about parenting and breastfeeding, but there are many things about your baby that you just can't learn from a book. What works for one baby may not work for another. Always trust your instincts in caring for your child—they are usually right! You will soon learn how your own special baby likes to be held, nursed, rocked, comforted, and entertained. The most important thing you can do for your baby during these early weeks is to follow his lead and make his life as pleasurable as possible.

Mature Milk

Your milk will start to change from colostrum to mature milk in about 3 to 4 days after the delivery, usually about the time you get home from the hospital. Mature milk is pale white or bluish in color and may look watery and thin. It will make your breasts feel fuller. The time when your milk "comes in" is different for every woman, but it depends on how often your baby has been nursing and how much colostrum he has been taking. It also depends on your body's own reaction to the birth.

The makeup of mature milk changes as your baby nurses—the milk your baby gets at the beginning of a feeding is different from the milk he gets at the end of the feeding. As your baby nurses, your milk increases in fat and calories. The milk your baby gets when he first latches on is called *foremilk*. **Foremilk** is watery and satisfies your baby's thirst. After a few minutes of sucking, *hindmilk* is released. **Hindmilk** has more fat and is more like heavy cream. Hindmilk satisfies your baby's hunger and gives him the calories he needs to gain weight.

Nursing Your Baby at Home

About the time your mature milk comes in, your baby's appetite will begin to increase. It is important to follow your baby's lead and feed him whenever he wants to nurse. This means nursing him when he shows signs of hunger or the need for comforting. During the first few days at home, some babies may nurse often and well, while others may be more interested in sleeping. Let your baby nurse for at least 10 minutes on each breast to make sure he is getting the calorie-rich hindmilk. Let him decide when he is finished with the first breast and is ready to switch. The longer he nurses on one breast, the more rich hindmilk he receives. Another nice benefit of mature milk is that it makes your baby feel calm and relaxed.

Once your mature milk comes in, your baby should nurse every 2 to 3 hours, or at least 8 to 12 times every 24 hours. Nursing your baby every 2 to 3 hours helps get your milk flowing and gives you a good milk supply. By feeding your baby when he shows signs of hunger he will learn to satisfy his own appetite. However, remember that if he sleeps for more than 4 hours you will need to wake him for a feeding. A good nursing session should last about 10 to 20 minutes on each breast, or 15 to 30 minutes on one breast if he nurses on only one side. However, some babies enjoy taking their time and may nurse for up to 45 minutes or longer, which is also normal.

Offering Both Breasts

Try to offer your baby both breasts at each feeding. Once your baby is latched on and positioned well, there is no reason to set a time limit for the feeding. Let him nurse from the first breast until he comes off on his own, either by pulling off or becoming sleepy. Then burp him and offer him the second breast. He may nurse longer, shorter, or not at all from the other breast. Just remember that once your mature milk comes in, it is more important that he nurse well on one breast (so he gets enough rich hindmilk) than to try to make him take the other breast if he is not interested. Begin the next feeding with the breast he took the *least* milk from at the last feeding. To help you remember, you can make a note in the "Baby's Feeding and Diaper Log" beginning on PAGE 38. You will soon be able to tell on your own which breast to start with at the next feeding, since the breast your baby took the least milk from will feel fuller than the other breast.

Cluster Feeding

During the early weeks of nursing, your baby may not show signs of hunger at the exact 2-hour or 3-hour periods that some new parents expect. Your baby may want to nurse more often at certain times of the day (usually during the evening) and may go longer between feedings at other times. This nursing pattern is called **cluster feeding** and is actually very common for most breastfed babies. The length of feedings as well as the time between feedings is different for every baby. Breastfed babies may nurse as often as every hour or as infrequently as every 3 to 4 hours, and still be healthy and grow. Remember that breast milk is easily digested, and babies' appetites change from day to day. It is more important to focus on the entire number of feedings in a 24-hour period, than the time between feedings. **Remember, the best way to tell if your baby is getting enough nourishment from breast milk is to check the number of wet and soiled diapers and amount weight gain.**

Most babies who cluster feed in the beginning naturally begin to go longer between feedings. They develop more regular feeding patterns as their digestive systems mature and they become better at getting milk from the breast. Remember, too, that babies nurse for comfort as well as for food. It is perfectly fine to nurse your baby if he seems fussy, even if it has been only 10 to 20 minutes since he last nursed. During these early days, nursing offers your newborn a great source of comfort and security when he becomes overwhelmed with his new environment.

Nighttime Feedings

Because newborns grow so rapidly and breast milk is quickly digested, it is normal for your baby to wake up at night and want to nurse. Also, your breasts can become engorged and uncomfortable if you wait too long between feedings. It may take a few weeks before your baby figures out the difference between night and day and starts sleeping for longer periods at night. **Just remember that during the first 4 weeks, if your baby is sleeping for longer than 4 hours, it is necessary to wake him for a feeding.**

To make nighttime feedings easier during these early weeks, you can have your newborn sleep in a cradle or bassinet next to your bed, or tuck him in bed beside you. If you choose to have your baby in your bed, there is no need to worry about rolling over on him. Under normal healthy conditions, mothers can sense their babies' presence even while sleeping. Just place your baby between you and the wall or a guardrail so that he is safely and securely on the bed. Do not allow your baby to sleep on a waterbed or with soft pillows, stuffed animals, or comforters. Your newborn's neck muscles are not yet strong enough to lift his own head if it becomes buried and he is unable to breath. With time, as your baby's tummy grows and his nursing pattern becomes more regular, he will begin to sleep for longer stretches at night—and so will you!

Elimination Patterns

During the early days, your baby's body is getting used to functioning on its own, and looking inside his diapers is one way to check his overall health. A sudden or unusual change in diaper contents or elimination patterns can be an important sign of a medical problem. **One of the best ways to tell if your baby is getting all the nutrition he needs is to keep track of wet and soiled diapers.** Remember, what goes in must come out! A sudden decrease in wet or soiled diapers may be a sign that your baby is not getting enough breast milk—and he could possibly become dehydrated. Using the "Baby's Feeding and Diaper Log," beginning on PAGE 38, will help you easily keep track of your baby's wet and soiled diapers for the first week.

Wet Diapers. Once your mature milk comes, your newborn's wet diapers will begin to increase. **He should have at least 6 to 8 wet diapers per day by Day 5.** His urine should continue to be pale yellow to almost clear in color. If your baby is having fewer than 6 wet diapers in a 24-hour period by Day 5, alert your baby's doctor—especially if your newborn is showing any signs of dehydration (see "Signs of Dehydration" on PAGE 35).

Soiled Diapers. When the meconium has passed (after the second or third day), you will begin to see *transitional stools*. This is when your baby's poops begin to *transition*, or change, from greenish-black to greenish-brown, and then to greenish-yellow in color. These transitional stools may be loose, unformed, and sometimes seedy in texture. After about 3 to 4 days of transitional stools, as your baby receives more of the high-fat hindmilk, his stools will become golden yellow in color, and mustard-like in texture. They may sometimes be seedy, curdly, loose, or even watery. Occasionally, babies have a watery gush called an *explosive stool*, which is normal and should not be confused with diarrhea. Because breast milk has a natural laxative effect, the stools of breastfed babies are softer and more frequent than those of formula-fed infants. They also have a milder odor. Still, during the first few weeks, many babies sometimes have to strain to pass a stool—even when the stool is soft or liquid. This problem is usually due to an immature digestive system and passes with time.

The number of stools per day varies among newborns. **But generally, after the meconium has passed and your mature milk has come in, your newborn should have at least 2 to 5 soiled diapers per day.** Some babies have a stool immediately after every breastfeeding session. But as the weeks go on, and your baby's digestive system matures, his stools may become less frequent and more regular. Within a month, he may have only 1 or 2 stools in an entire week. This is not uncommon as long as your baby is healthy and growing. While these changes are normal, you should contact your baby's doctor if you see any sudden, unusual changes in your baby's stools, especially if your baby has other symptoms such as fever, lethargy, or irritability. See "Warnings Signs for Baby" on PAGE 59.

Growth Spurts

At times, you may notice that your baby seems to be breastfeeding well, and then all of a sudden he becomes extra hungry and seems to want to nurse all the time. **Because babies grow so quickly in such a short period of time, they go through occasional *growth spurts*, or sudden periods of rapid growth.** During these periods your baby may be hungrier and fussier than normal and you may think that you are not making enough milk. But actually the opposite is true. The fact that your baby is nursing more often increases your milk supply to meet his growing needs.

Growth spurts usually last for 2 to 3 days, or until your milk supply catches up to your baby's increased needs. After the growth spurt, your baby's feeding pattern will begin to space out once again. Growth spurts are fairly predictable and usually happen around 2 weeks, 6 weeks, 3 months, and 6 months of age.

Is Your Baby Getting Enough?

Nursing mothers often worry about whether their babies are "getting enough," especially since they have no way of measuring exactly how much breast milk their babies are taking in. During the first few weeks, it is sometimes difficult to tell, especially for first-time mothers. However, after the first month or so, you will know that your baby is getting enough to eat by the way he is nursing and the way his body is filling out and growing. Breastfed babies eat about 2½ ounces of breast milk each day for every pound they weigh. (So a 10-pound baby would eat about 25 ounces of breast milk per day.) Here are the signs to look for in the first few weeks to ensure that your breastfeeding baby is "getting enough":

Day 1 through Day 3

- Your baby is offered a feeding of *colostrum* every 1½ to 3 hours around the clock, and is nursing at least 10 to 12 times every 24 hours.
- While receiving *colostrum*, your baby passes *meconium*, the greenish-black, sticky, tarlike first stools.
- While receiving *colostrum*, your baby has at least 1 to 2 wet diapers every 24 hours. His urine should be pale yellow to clear in color.

Once your mature milk comes in:

- Your baby nurses every 2 to 3 hours or at least 8 to 12 times every 24 hours.
- Your baby has passed the *meconium* and has at least 2 to 5 soiled diapers every 24 hours.
- Your baby has at least 6 to 8 wet diapers every 24 hours. His urine should be pale yellow to clear in color.
- You feel a tugging (not pain) at your nipple and areola as your baby latches on.
- You hear your baby sucking and swallowing, and his cheeks are rounded.
- Your breasts feel full before a feeding and softer after the feeding.
- Your baby seems satisfied or sleepy after each feeding, not fussy.
- Your baby is gaining 4 to 7 ounces per week, or at least 1 pound per month.
- Your baby appears healthy, has good color and skin tone, is filling out and growing in length and head circumference, and is alert and active.

If you feel that your baby is not getting enough breast milk, talk to your doctor or a lactation specialist. Someone with expert knowledge of breastfeeding can help you solve any problems you may have while making sure your baby is getting enough fluids and calories.

Signs of Dehydration

When a baby becomes dehydrated (loses body fluids), it is usually due to diarrhea or vomiting from an illness. However, a healthy baby who is not getting enough breast milk can also become dehydrated. Since tiny babies need more fluids and use them more quickly than adults, the lack of fluids in a small baby is more harmful than in an adult. This is why newborns who do not wake up on their own at night to nurse need to be awakened—even if they are not showing signs of hunger. An entire night without a feeding is far too long for a newborn to go without fluids. When a baby becomes seriously short of fluids, his body is not able to function properly. It is very important to be aware of the signs of dehydration. Contact your baby's doctor immediately if you notice any of the following symptoms in your newborn:

- fewer than 6 wet diapers every 24 hours after the 4th day
- fewer than 2 bowel movements every 24 hours after the 4th day
- slower than normal weight gain
- red or pink "brick dust" appearance on the diaper (uric acid crystals)
- dark-colored urine
- soft spot on the top of the head (fontanel) appears sunken
- refuses to nurse and has missed 2 feedings in a row
- fever, vomiting, or diarrhea
- a sudden increase in sleepiness and difficulty waking
- unusual irritability or crying
- a decreased amount of tears when crying
- dry mouth and lips
- cool, discolored hands and feet
- loose, wrinkly skin
- sunken eyes

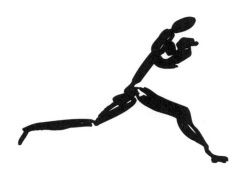

Keeping Track of Your Breastfeeding Baby

The best way to tell if your baby is getting enough breast milk is by counting the number of feedings and wet and soiled diapers. The following table gives you an overview of Week 1 and shows you how many feedings and wet and soiled diapers your baby should have each day for the first week:

Overview of Week 1			
DAY	FEEDINGS	WET DIAPERS	SOILED DIAPERS
Day 1	10–12	1 pale yellow	1 tarry, greenish-black
Day 2	10–12	1–2 pale yellow	1–2 tarry, greenish-black
Day 3	10–12	2–4 pale yellow	2 loose, greenish-brown
Day 4	8–12	4–6 pale yellow	2–5 loose, greenish-yellow
Day 5	8–12	6–8 pale yellow	2–5 soft, golden yellow
Day 6	8–12	6–8 pale yellow	2–5 soft, golden yellow
Day 7	8–12	6–8 pale yellow	2–5 soft, golden yellow

The **"Baby's Feeding and Diaper Log,"** beginning on the next page, will help you keep track of your baby for the first week. The shaded boxes show you the minimum number of feedings and wet and soiled diapers your baby should have each day. Keep track throughout the day by putting an "X" in the correct boxes. At the end of the day, there should be an "X" in all the shaded boxes. It is fine if your baby has more than what is indicated, but make sure he has at least the minimum number. Remember, one day is a 24-hour period. If any of the shaded boxes does **not** have an "X" in it for more than one day, call your baby's doctor. Your baby may not be getting enough breast milk.

The following is an example of how to fill in the log for Day 1:

An Example of Day 1													
DAY 1								**DATE:** *January 3*					
GOAL	1	2	3	4	5	6	7	8	9	10	11	12	TOTALS
10–12 Feedings	X	X	X	X	X	X	X	X	X	X	X		11
1 Wet Diaper	X pale yellow												1
1 Soiled Diaper	X tarry greenish-black	X											2
Notes: ***Baby nursed right after birth!***													

Baby's Feeding and Diaper Log

Birth Date _____ Birth Weight _____

Time _____ Discharge Weight _____

WEEK 1

DAY 1	DATE:												
GOAL	1	2	3	4	5	6	7	8	9	10	11	12	TOTALS
10–12 Feedings													
1 Wet Diaper	pale yellow												
1 Soiled Diaper	tarry greenish-black												
Notes:													

DAY 2	DATE:												
GOAL	1	2	3	4	5	6	7	8	9	10	11	12	TOTALS
10–12 Feedings													
1–2 Wet Diapers	pale yellow												
1–2 Soiled Diapers	tarry greenish-black												
Notes:													

DAY 3   DATE:

GOAL	1	2	3	4	5	6	7	8	9	10	11	12	TOTALS
10–12 Feedings													
2–4 Wet Diapers	pale yellow	pale yellow											
2 Soiled Diapers	loose greenish-brown	loose greenish-brown											

Notes:

DAY 4   DATE:

GOAL	1	2	3	4	5	6	7	8	9	10	11	12	TOTALS
8–12 Feedings													
4–6 Wet Diapers	pale yellow	pale yellow	pale yellow	pale yellow									
2–5 Soiled Diapers	loose greenish-yellow	loose greenish-yellow											

Notes:

DAY 5   DATE:

GOAL	1	2	3	4	5	6	7	8	9	10	11	12	TOTALS
8–12 Feedings													
6–8 Wet Diapers	pale yellow	pale yellow	pale yellow	pale yellow	pale yellow	pale yellow							
2–5 Soiled Diapers	soft golden yellow	soft golden yellow											

Notes:

DAY 6													DATE:
GOAL	1	2	3	4	5	6	7	8	9	10	11	12	TOTALS
8–12 Feedings													
6–8 Wet Diapers	pale yellow	pale yellow	pale yellow	pale yellow	pale yellow	pale yellow							
2–5 Soiled Diapers	soft golden yellow	soft golden yellow											

Notes:

DAY 7													DATE:
GOAL	1	2	3	4	5	6	7	8	9	10	11	12	TOTALS
8–12 Feedings													
6–8 Wet Diapers	pale yellow	pale yellow	pale yellow	pale yellow	pale yellow	pale yellow							
2–5 Soiled Diapers	soft golden yellow	soft golden yellow											

Notes:

END OF WEEK 1

Baby's weight at the end of Week 1: _____

Questions for the baby's doctor or lactation specialist: _____

_____

_____

_____

Breastfeeding and Sexuality

As new parents it may be more difficult to find the time or energy to be intimate with each other during the early days. But sex after a baby can be very special, as the warmth and love you feel for your baby carries over into your feelings for each other. A new mother's feelings about being sexual with her partner are different for every woman. Some new mothers find that they are not as interested in sex as they were before the baby was born, while others have an increased sexual desire.

There are many reasons why a new mother may be less interested in sex. The hormone *estrogen*, which influences a woman's sex drive, is produced in lower amounts after giving birth. This may cause a decreased sexual desire in some new mothers. But this is only temporary and usually improves once a woman's menstrual cycle begins again. Sometimes being close to your baby all day long lessens your desire for physical contact with your partner. You may also worry that lovemaking may be painful or that you may get pregnant again. But one of the main reasons mothers lose their desire for sex is due to pure exhaustion. It is understandable that a mother who spends 24 hours a day caring for her baby may see 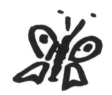 sex quite differently from her partner who spends most of his time outside the home. It is important to share your feelings with your partner and help him understand why you are feeling less of a desire for sex.

Most new mothers can usually resume sexual intercourse about 6 weeks after a vaginal delivery or 8 to 10 weeks after a cesarean section. You may have some vaginal dryness during lovemaking, due to the lower estrogen levels in your body. Using a water soluble lubricant such as K-Y Jelly may be helpful. Breastfeeding does not have to make your breasts off-limits to your partner. Your breasts may feel tender during the early days of nursing, but this is only temporary. Nursing before you make love should help with breast tenderness. Also, it is not unusual for a woman's breasts to spray milk, especially during orgasm, since the same hormone that is released during sex (oxytocin) also stimulates the milk-ejection reflex.

Sometimes women with highly sensitive breasts may experience sexual arousal on occasion as they nurse their babies. This is completely normal and certainly nothing to feel guilty about. Because of the strong hormonal connection between breastfeeding and sex, your body is responding naturally to your baby's sucking. But most often, the physical sensations of breastfeeding are felt as an overall sense of well-being and great tenderness toward your baby.

Making time to be intimate with your partner on a regular basis will help keep your relationship strong. Choose a time when your baby usually sleeps to be intimate. Plan ahead so that you can be rested and are able to give lovemaking your full attention.

Breastfeeding in Public

Many women nurse their babies wherever they happen to be without anyone ever noticing what they are doing. The more you nurse, the easier it gets. If you feel a little shy about nursing in front of other people, you can excuse yourself and go into another room. Or you can start your baby nursing in another room and then rejoin the group. Usually, the only time your breasts may be exposed is when your baby first latches on.

Once your baby is latched on, it is easier to keep your breasts covered. In public places, you can usually find an out-of-the-way spot, or you can have a companion block you from public view. Most people will respect your privacy. Wearing simple, loose-fitting clothing makes it easier for you to nurse in public.

What to Wear

- Two-piece outfits with loose-fitting shirts are the most practical. You can lift the shirt from the bottom up so the baby can get to your breast. The rest of the fabric from the shirt will drape over the baby's head and cover any exposed skin.
- To protect your middle from being exposed, cut slits at breast level in a form fitting T-shirt or tank top. Then wear it *under* a loose-fitting shirt. When you lift the outer shirt, the T-shirt or tank top stays in place, giving you extra coverage.
- Wear shirts, blouses, or sweaters with buttons down the front and unbutton them from the bottom up, rather than the top down.
- Drape a lightweight blanket or shawl over your shoulder and your baby while you nurse.
- Try using a baby sling. While you are nursing, your baby stays hidden behind the fabric of the sling and appears to be sleeping.
- Wear nursing bras with cups that are easy to unfasten with one hand, which makes it easier to get started at the breast.
- Tops with small prints are good at hiding leaking and spit-up stains.
- You can also purchase special clothing for nursing mothers, with hidden openings at the breasts, at maternity shops, department stores, or from breastfeeding catalogs.

Where to Go

- In a public place, find an out-of-the-way bench or private area.
- In a restaurant, sit at a corner table with your back to the room.
- At the mall, you can usually use a fitting room in a department store.
- If there is no comfortable place for you to nurse in public, you can always nurse in your car or a restroom.
- Many public places are now providing special areas for mothers to nurse—look for them in your community.

Getting Started

One of the best ways not to draw attention to yourself while you are nursing is to know your baby's hunger signs. Feed him before he is overly hungry and making a fuss. He will latch on more easily, and you won't have people looking your way. Remember, the only time your breast may be exposed is when your baby first latches on. This is usually not a problem if your baby is covered with a blanket or hidden behind your shirt or a baby sling. If you are sitting on a bench or a chair without arms, you can use your diaper bag or a folded blanket or coat to bring the baby up to breast level while you nurse. Your outing will be much more enjoyable if you don't go home with sore nipples or a cramp in your arm or back because of poor positioning.

Breastfeeding Laws

Many states have passed laws giving women the right to breastfeed their babies in public places. There is also a similar federal law allowing breastfeeding on federal property. While women have occasionally made the news for breastfeeding in public places, in the end, the nursing mother is usually the one who receives an apology. Because the benefits of breastfeeding are becoming more widely recognized, the general public is beginning to accept it as a natural part of life. Besides, it's good for the reputations of businesses and public facilities to meet the needs of breastfeeding families.

Thousands of American mothers nurse their babies every day—at parks, shopping centers, malls, or other public places—and most people either don't notice or don't mind. Some people will even look their way and smile approvingly. Remember that mothers all over the world nurse their babies wherever they may be and think nothing of it, because it is their way of life.

If you do happen to run into someone who does not approve of your breastfeeding in public, be polite and let the person know that it is your right to give your baby the best nutrition possible—and be proud of yourself!

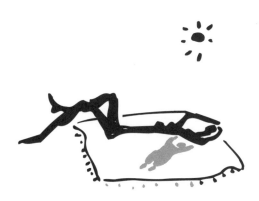

CHAPTER 3

Solving Breastfeeding Problems

Breastfeeding may go smoothly right from the start, or you may run into some difficulties along the way. When difficulties do occur, it is usually during the first 6 weeks after birth. But with proper attention, most problems can be prevented or easily treated. This chapter will help you recognize possible problems and know when to call for help. With the right information and a little help, a mother who is determined to breastfeed can get through most challenges. And usually, the sooner you get help, the easier the problem is to resolve.

Identifying Common Newborn Problems

Sucking Problems

Some newborns have problems sucking and are not able to suck at the breast for various reasons. These babies are able to latch on to the breast, but because their suction is weak they slide off while nursing. Most of the time, these babies are not using their tongues correctly or may be sucking on their tongues rather than the breast, a habit that may have developed in the womb. Some infants with sucking problems may be **tongue-tied**. This is when the **frenulum**, the membrane that attaches the tongue to the floor of the mouth, is very short. This makes it difficult for the baby to stick his tongue out far enough to grab the underside of his mother's breast. Some babies may have a very **high palate** (roof of the mouth) or a **small lower jaw** that makes it difficult for them to latch on to the breast. In all cases of sucking difficulties, it is best to get help from a lactation specialist or someone who has experience helping babies with sucking problems. You may need to give your baby pumped breast milk until he is able to suck on his own. With patience, determination, and the right help, most babies with sucking problems are eventually able to get all their nourishment at the breast.

Nipple Confusion

It is recommended that you wait at least 3 to 4 weeks, or until breastfeeding is going well, before offering your baby artificial nipples (bottles or pacifiers). This will lessen the chance of the artificial nipple confusing your baby. Sucking at the breast takes a little more skill and effort than sucking a bottle. When a baby sucks at the breast, he needs to draw the milk out of his mother's nipple using an active sucking motion. Sucking a bottle is easier for a baby because the milk just drips into his mouth. Artificial nipples given in the early days may interfere with your baby's learning process and may affect your milk supply.

Lip Blisters

During the early months of breastfeeding, many newborns get blisters on the center of their upper lip. These lip blisters are normal and are caused by active sucking at the breast. Lip blisters are not a medical problem and do not cause discomfort to your baby. They usually go away by themselves without any treatment, and sometimes they even seem to disappear between feedings.

Jaundice

Jaundice is a condition that causes the skin and whites of the eyes to yellow. Jaundice is fairly common in newborns and is usually nothing to worry about. Breastfeeding often (at least 10 to 12 times every 24 hours) in the first few days will help prevent jaundice. Many cases of jaundice do not need to be treated; however a doctor should carefully monitor your baby until it passes.

While in the womb, a baby gets oxygen from his red blood cells. After birth, the baby's lungs give him oxygen, so the extra red blood cells are no longer needed. As the extra red blood cells are broken down, a by-product called **bilirubin**, a yellow bile pigment, is released into the blood. The bilirubin is then processed by the liver and passed though the baby's stools (poops). Sometimes a newborn's immature liver cannot process the bilirubin as fast as it is being produced, so it builds up in the blood and jaundice results. Increasing the number of feedings will increase the number of stools and help carry the bilirubin out of his body. This type of jaundice is called **normal (physiologic) jaundice** and it often clears up within a week or two as the baby's liver becomes more efficient, usually without any treatment.

Another type of jaundice known as **abnormal (pathological) jaundice** is rare and develops within the first 24 hours after birth. This usually occurs because of incompatible blood types of the mother and baby, or a liver-related problem. In the case of abnormal jaundice, treatment is usually necessary to bring down the bilirubin level. A treatment called **phototherapy** is usually prescribed. The newborn is placed under special fluorescent lights called *bili-lights* for 24 to 48 hours. These special lights lower the level of bilirubin in the blood by breaking it down. Although the baby's skin may still be yellow for a few days, once the bilirubin starts to decrease, no further treatment is necessary.

In most cases of jaundice, it is very important to continue to breastfeed as often as possible to increase the amount of the baby's stools, which is necessary to eliminate the buildup of bilirubin. To check for jaundice, firmly press your thumb on your baby's nose or thigh, then release. If the skin is yellow-colored, contact your baby's doctor.

Spitting Up

Spitting up is very normal for newborns, especially during the early days. Although it may look like a whole meal on your shirt, usually it is not more than a few teaspoons. Some babies spit up because they are getting too much milk too quickly and are taking in air along with it. Some excited eaters just become too full and their tiny tummies have no choice but to send some milk back up. Some babies spit up a small amount after every meal. This is usually due to an immature digestive system and passes with time. By about 6 to 7 months, when your baby is able to sit upright, gravity will keep the milk down and he will spit up much less. In the meantime, be prepared by dressing for the occasion and always have a burp cloth or towel handy. Here are some more helpful tips:

- Burp your baby before switching sides, and then again at the end of each feeding.
- Hold your baby as upright as possible while nursing. After each feeding, try to keep him upright for 20 to 30 minutes. (You can wear your baby in an upright position in a baby sling or carrier.)
- Handle your baby gently after each feeding and try not to bounce or rock him for at least 30 minutes.

Vomiting

Vomiting is a stronger type of spitting up in which the milk usually ends up farther away from the baby's mouth. Vomiting is usually not a serious problem as long as the baby is healthy and growing. However, **projectile vomiting**, when the milk shoots forcefully through the air and ends up a few feet away, can be caused by an infection, a virus, or pyloric stenosis. **Pyloric stenosis** is a condition in which the pyloric valve between the stomach and the small intestine doesn't open properly and the milk cannot pass through, so it stays in the stomach. As the stomach contracts, it causes the milk to shoot back up through the *esophagus* (the tube in the throat) and out of the mouth. This condition can usually be identified within the first 2 months. If your baby is projectile vomiting, it is necessary to call your baby's doctor as soon as possible. Your baby may be losing most of the milk he is taking in, and if untreated he could lose weight and become dehydrated. Pyloric stenosis is corrected with a simple operation which permanently loosens the pyloric valve. If your baby is vomiting a bright-green bile liquid, or vomits while showing other signs of illness such as refusing to eat, diarrhea, fever, unusual crying, or slow weight gain, contact your baby's doctor.

Gastroesophageal Reflux (GER)

In some cases, spitting up or projectile vomiting can be a sign of a medical condition called **gastroesophageal reflux (GER)**. A baby with GER may cry and scream when he tries to nurse. And when he does nurse, he may gag, choke, or have difficulty swallowing. With this condition, the muscle at the opening of the stomach opens at the wrong time, allowing milk and food to come back up into the esophagus. Also, stomach acids, which usually stay in the stomach to digest food, may enter the esophagus. This causes the esophagus tissues to become inflamed and makes eating very uncomfortable. If your baby is showing signs of GER, contact your baby's doctor for treatment.

Diarrhea

Breastfed babies rarely have diarrhea because certain ingredients in breast milk seem to destroy much of the bacteria that causes diarrhea. It is quite normal for breastfed babies to have very soft, loose, sometimes watery stools, but they should not be mistaken for diarrhea. However, older breastfed babies sometimes do get diarrhea. If your baby is having a large number of stools (12 to 16 in a 24-hour period) or has stools that are liquid, have a bad odor, or have specks of blood or mucus, he most likely has diarrhea. If symptoms don't improve within 24 hours, or your baby does not want to nurse, is vomiting, crying unusually, or has a fever, contact your baby's doctor. If your baby is willing to nurse, keep breastfeeding. Nursing frequently will prevent dehydration.

Constipation

Breastfed babies usually don't have a problem with constipation. Although, it is normal for newborns to sometimes have difficulty passing a stool. At times, a baby may seem uncomfortable and cry, grunt, or groan as he passes a stool. This is usually because of his immature digestive system and not constipation. Constipation is when a baby has hard, dry stools, possibly containing streaks of blood, and a full uncomfortable tummy. If your baby is only being breastfed, he will most likely not become constipated. But if you feel that your baby is having a problem with constipation, call your baby's doctor.

Colic

Colic is when a baby has regular, long periods of very loud scream-like crying for no reason that you can see. The cause of colic is unknown, but some experts think it is due to an immature digestive and/or nervous system. Colic can appear in either breastfed or formula-fed babies. It is believed that it is better to breastfeed a baby who has colic, since breast milk is much easier to digest.

A baby with colic usually has screaming fits every day about the same time, often during the late afternoon or early evening. Sometimes a baby with colic will pull his knees up, clench his fists in agony, and seem to be in physical pain. This behavior generally begins at about 3 to 4 weeks of age. A crying session may continue for up to 3 to 5 hours or more, day after day. The good news is that babies usually outgrow these screaming fits between 6 weeks and 3 months of age—without any ill effects. There is no known cure for colic, except time.

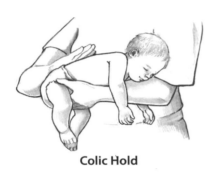

Colic Hold

Sometimes a baby may appear to have colic because something the mother is eating may be causing the same symptoms. Cow's milk products, eggs, citrus fruits, nuts, gas-inducing foods (such as cabbage, broccoli, and dried beans), and caffeine may cause colic symptoms in some babies, especially if there is a family history of allergies. If after eating any of these foods you notice your baby is having colic symptoms, try avoiding the food for a week to see if there is an improvement in your baby. However, if you are finding it necessary to avoid all dairy products, you may need to talk to a dietitian to help you plan an appropriate diet to make sure you are getting enough calcium from other foods or dietary supplements. Here are some suggestions for a baby with colic:

- Try the *colic hold:* lay your baby tummy-down on your arm with his head at your elbow and your hand cupped between his legs. Hold him against your body and raise his head so it is slightly higher than his feet. This position puts pressure on the stomach, sometimes making the baby more comfortable.
- Feed your baby smaller, more frequent meals to avoid overfeeding, and burp him often.
- Try nursing on only one breast at each feeding to make sure that your baby is getting enough rich hindmilk and less foremilk, which contains more lactose and may give him gas.

48

- To relieve gas, lay your baby on his back and gently rotate his legs as if he were riding a bicycle.
- Carry your baby around in a sling or baby carrier.
- Swaddle your baby with a blanket and pat or rub his back.
- Lay your baby on your chest so he can feel your heartbeat.
- Give your baby a warm bath or put a warm washcloth on his tummy.
- Rhythmically rock your baby in a cradle or in your arms.
- Play "white noise" such as the hum of a fan or a vacuum cleaner, or play nature sounds or soft music.
- Try to identify and eliminate foods in your diet that may be causing colic symptoms.
- When it becomes too overwhelming, take a break and give your baby to your partner or another caregiver. Sometimes just a fresh set of arms may calm your baby.

Whatever the cause of colic, calm and gentle handling is what your baby needs. Sometimes with a colicky baby, nothing that you do seems to help. But as upsetting as colic is for parents, it is important to accept it as a passing phase and try to handle it as calmly as possible. Help your baby through this difficult time by responding to his pain. He doesn't know why he is feeling this way any more than you do. Comfort him and let him know that you are there for him. Be sure to mention the crying pattern (when, how long, how often, and how intense) to your baby's doctor to rule out any medical problem. Any sudden crying spells in a baby who has not shown colic symptoms could indicate illness.

Biting

Sometimes, as babies begin to get their teeth (beginning at about 3 months), they may try to bite your nipple during a nursing session. The biting most often happens at the end of a feeding when your baby is already full. A baby cannot bite while he is nursing because his tongue is covering his bottom teeth. Babies usually bite because they are teething or just feeling playful. When this happens, remove your baby from your breast and firmly say, "no." If he is still hungry, offer the breast again. If the biting continues, take him off the breast for several minutes this time. Your baby will eventually learn that biting is not acceptable and brings an end to breastfeeding. If you think your baby is biting because he is teething, watch him as he nurses. As soon as he stops sucking, take him off the breast quickly so he doesn't have a chance to bite.

Nursing Strike

A nursing strike is when your baby has been nursing well for a few months and then suddenly he doesn't want to nurse. Nursing strikes most often happen with babies older than 3 months of age. A baby on a nursing strike may seem fine, but when offered the breast he may cry and turn away. Usually the baby is trying to let you know that something is bothering him. A nursing strike usually lasts just a few days but may continue for up to a week or two. If your baby is on a nursing strike, it is normal to feel frustrated, especially if your baby is unhappy. But it is important not to feel guilty or that you have done something wrong. Try to determine the cause, if you can. But often times the cause is never known. Some possible causes of a nursing strike may include:

- a stuffy nose, cold, sore throat, or other illness
- teething, cold sore, ear infection, thrush
- the frequent use of bottles or pacifiers
- a forceful let-down reflex
- a response to the mother's reaction to being bitten
- stress or over-stimulation in the baby
- a sudden change in the household or in the family's daily routine
- mother using a new perfume, lotion, soap, or spray
- mother taking a new medication
- pain in a certain nursing position due to an injury or soreness from an immunization

The following suggestions may be helpful in getting your baby back to the breast:

- Try nursing when your baby is drowsy or asleep, especially at night. This is the most common and effective way to end a nursing strike. Some babies will begin nursing at night several days before they return to daytime feedings.
- Before trying to nurse, pump for a few minutes to get the milk flowing.
- Try different nursing positions. Nurse while lying down or in a quiet, dark room.
- You can also try nursing while standing, walking, or gently bouncing.
- Give your baby lots of skin-to-skin contact, not only while nursing but at other times as well.
- Try nursing while you take a warm bath together.
- If your baby becomes upset while trying to nurse, stop and try to calm him before trying again. You don't want your baby to think of nursing as unpleasant.

During a nursing strike, your breasts may become uncomfortably full as the milk builds up. It is important to express your breast milk as often as your baby was nursing to keep up your milk supply and relieve engorgement. If you will be pumping several times per day, you may want to look into renting a hospital-grade breast pump. While waiting for a nursing strike to end, you can use a dropper, spoon, cup, or bottle to give your baby your breast milk. If you choose to use a bottle, use a newborn or slow-flow nipple so that the baby still has to work to get milk from the bottle. Older babies will usually just eat more solid foods. It is important to offer the breast, but try not to push it. If a baby feels pressured, it may take longer for him to get over the strike. Stay calm and give him plenty of attention.

Most nursing strikes do end happily. Patience is the most important tool in getting through a nursing strike. Some babies who have been on strike for a week or more may just start breastfeeding again as if nothing had happened. Others slowly come back to the breast as their noses clear, their throats heal, or they get their confidence back. Whatever the cause may be, if a strike lasts more than 2 or 3 days, it is helpful to have the support of your doctor or a lactation specialist.

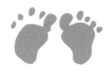

Managing Difficulties the Mother May Have

Nipple Tenderness

During the early days of breastfeeding, it is normal to have some nipple tenderness. You may feel a little discomfort each time you begin to nurse, as your baby draws the nipple and areola into his mouth. It may last only a few seconds and should disappear as soon as the nipple is positioned far back in the baby's mouth away from the friction of his tongue and gums. **This early nipple tenderness should pass once your mature milk comes in and your breasts go through a period of conditioning.** If there is continued pain after this initial discomfort, it is most likely because your baby is not latched on correctly. If this initial discomfort does not go away within a few days, or you feel pain throughout a feeding, contact a lactation specialist for help with proper positioning.

Sore Nipples

If tender nipples become sore after the initial latch-on discomfort, it usually means that your baby has not been latching on correctly. If a latch-on problem is not corrected quickly, your nipples may become cracked and painful. Here are some tips for preventing and treating sore nipples:

Preventing Sore Nipples:

- Make sure your baby is positioned correctly and has the nipple and a large part of the areola in his mouth. His lips should be turned outward.
- Breastfeed your baby frequently, at least every 2 to 3 hours during the day and every 3 to 4 hours at night.
- Offer both breasts at each feeding.
- Release the baby's suction before taking him off the breast by gently putting your finger into the corner of his mouth to break the suction.
- Gently pat your nipples dry after each feeding session.
- Begin each new feeding with the breast your baby took the *least* milk from at the last feeding.
- Avoid using anything other than plain warm water to wash your breasts and nipples.
- Wear cotton bras rather than synthetic ones (polyester, etc.).
- Change your nursing pads often. Avoid the ones with plastic liners because they prevent air circulation.

Treating Sore Nipples:

- Change to a position where the baby's jaws put pressure on other, less tender areas of the breast.
- Try not to miss feedings. Shorter more frequent feedings, every 1 to 2 hours, are easier on the nipples.
- Breastfeed on the least sore side first.
- Express a little breast milk to stimulate the let-down reflex, which makes the areola softer, the nipple more erect, and latch-on easier.
- Express a little breast milk onto the nipple and areola and let air-dry. Breast milk contains substances that help fight infection and promote healing.

- If there are cracks in the nipple skin, you can use 100% modified lanolin to soothe and moisturize the nipples and speed healing.
- If your bra or clothing feels uncomfortable against your nipples, you can use 100% modified lanolin and wear breast shells. Breast shells keep the fabric from rubbing against your nipples.
- Wear soft, natural-fiber clothing that feels smooth and comfortable against your nipples, and check to make sure there are no scratchy seams in your bra.
- Talk to your doctor about a pain reliever approved for breastfeeding mothers.
- If nipple cracking is more severe on one breast, you may want to use a breast pump on that side until you are comfortable breastfeeding again with that breast.
- If soreness continues, contact a lactation specialist to determine the cause.

Engorgement

A few days after the delivery, as colostrum changes to mature milk, your breasts may become uncomfortably full. Breast fullness is a normal condition and is caused by an increased supply of blood and fluid, as well as milk, in the breast tissue. Normal postpartum fullness usually eases up within 2 to 3 days. Engorgement develops if your baby does not take enough milk from your breasts. This usually happens when feedings are too far apart or missed. The breasts may become swollen and feel tender, hard, and painful. The skin on your breasts may look shiny and feel hot. Too much fullness can lead to swollen areolas and flat nipples, making it difficult for your baby to latch on. By breastfeeding often, and keeping the breasts as empty as possible, the engorgement should pass within 48 hours. **Remember, the more you nurse your baby, the less likely you are to become engorged.** If engorgement continues or is severe, and the following suggestions have not helped, contact a lactation specialist.

Preventing Engorgement:
- Breastfeed your baby often, at least every 2 to 3 hours during the day and every 3 to 4 hours at night.
- Begin each new feeding with the breast your baby took the *least* milk from at the last feeding.
- Offer both breasts at each feeding.
- Avoid pacifiers or bottles of water or formula.
- Express your breast milk to relieve fullness if you delay or miss a feeding.
- Wear a supportive bra that fits well. Avoid bras that have underwires or are too tight.

Treating Engorgement:
- Breastfeed your baby often, at least every 1 to 2 hours during the day and every 2 to 3 hours at night.
- Begin each new feeding with the breast your baby took the *least* milk from at the last feeding.
- Offer both breasts at each feeding.
- Apply warm, moist compresses to the breast for a few minutes just before nursing (such as a warm, moist washcloth).
- Express just enough breast milk to soften the areolas and make the nipples soft

before nursing. (Do not overdo it, as pumping more than necessary defeats the purpose by stimulating milk production.)

- As your baby nurses on your breast, gently massage it from the chest wall toward the nipple.
- Apply cold compresses to your breasts between feedings to reduce swelling, relieve pain, and help slow the engorgement process. (Zip-lock bags filled with frozen peas wrapped in a wet washcloth work well.)
- Take a warm shower just before a feeding session.
- Talk to your doctor about a pain reliever approved for breastfeeding mothers.
- Some nursing mothers find relief from engorgement by wearing chilled green cabbage leaves inside their nursing bras between feedings. To use this simple home remedy, wash cabbage leaves and store in a Zip-lock bag in the refrigerator. When ready to use, lightly crumple a whole leaf in your hand (to crush the veins), cut out a hole for your nipple, and place over your breast, inside your bra. Change leaves about every two hours (or when wilted) and repeat if necessary.

Leaking

Leaking most often happens during the early weeks of nursing. Leaking may occur unexpectedly between feedings or during the night. Sometimes, while your baby is nursing on one breast, the other breast may leak or squirt milk. Leaking is caused by the release of the hormone *oxytocin* which triggers the let-down reflex. Any suggestion that it is nursing time, such as full breasts, the sound of your baby's cry (or any baby's cry), or just thinking about your baby, can trigger a let-down—whether you're ready to nurse or not. Leaking may also occur when you delay or miss a feeding and your breasts become overly full. **Leaking usually eases up in the second month, once your baby's demand and your supply become more in tune.** In the meantime, here are some tips for leaking breasts:

- Wear nursing pads in your bra to absorb any leaking milk and be sure to change them often. Avoid the ones with plastic liners because they prevent air circulation.
- Wear washable, loose-style shirts with small prints to hide milk stains. Always take extra nursing pads and an extra bra and shirt when going out.
- Try not to delay feedings, but if you can't avoid it, express some milk when your breasts become overly full.
- While you are nursing from one breast, use a nursing pad or small towel to catch milk dripping from the other breast.
- Breastfeed before going to bed and sleep with a comfortable bra lined with nursing pads.
- Here is a way to stop inconvenient leaking: as you feel a let-down occurring, cross your arms in front of you, and with the palms of your hands apply pressure against your nipples for several seconds. (Use this technique only when necessary and only after your milk supply is fully established, since constant pressure on your breasts can cause plugged ducts.)

Plugged Ducts

Sometimes when milk gets backed up in the breast, a milk duct can become plugged. This usually happens because the breast was not emptied completely or there was continued pressure on one or more of the milk ducts. **When milk is not able to flow freely through the duct, it can become inflamed and plug up.** A plugged duct may look hard and lumpy and there may be a painful area on your breast that feels hot and tender. The basic treatment for a plugged duct is to keep the milk flowing by breastfeeding often and emptying the breasts as much as possible at each feeding. It is more important than ever to continue breastfeeding when you have a plugged duct. In fact, it is best to nurse on the affected side first when your baby is hungriest. His strong suck will actually help clear out the plug. Prompt and proper treatment of a plugged duct will usually prevent a breast infection (*mastitis*) from developing. Here are some tips for preventing and treating plugged ducts:

Preventing Plugged Ducts:

- Try not to delay or miss feedings. Nurse every 2 to 3 hours, emptying the breasts as completely as possible.
- Change your nursing position throughout the day to put pressure on different milk ducts at each feeding.
- Gently clean any dried milk blocking your nipple pores with a cotton ball and plain warm water.
- Hand express or pump just enough breast milk to relieve breast fullness.
- Avoid bras that have underwires or are too tight.
- Avoid putting pressure on your breasts with tight clothing, heavy shoulder bags, or infant carriers.

Treating Plugged Ducts:

- Nurse your baby more frequently around the clock.
- Apply warm, moist compresses to the breast for a few minutes just before breastfeeding (such as a warm, moist washcloth).
- Nurse on the affected side first so that your baby empties it as thoroughly as possible.
- Breastfeed in a different position. Aim your baby's chin in the direction of the plugged duct. The baby's suction will help release the plug.
- Gently massage the plugged duct downward toward the nipple while you are breastfeeding or while you are in the shower.
- If your baby does not empty the affected breast, hand express or pump the milk that is left.
- Between feedings use warm, moist compresses and massage to encourage the plug to travel down the duct.
- Keep pressure off the plugged duct. Make sure your bra and clothing do not put pressure on your breasts in any way.
- Avoid sleeping on your stomach which puts pressure on your breasts.
- Avoid using nipple shields.
- Get extra rest and eliminate extra activities.
- Make sure you are eating a nutritious diet and getting plenty of fluids.
- If you are experiencing plugged ducts frequently, consult a lactation specialist to check your positioning and latch-on technique.

Mastitis

If a plugged duct is not treated, it can develop into a breast infection known as *mastitis.* If the tender area on your breast becomes more and more painful, and you develop flu-like symptoms such as a high fever, achiness, headache, fatigue, chills, and sometimes nausea and vomiting, you most likely have mastitis. Usually, only a certain area of the breast is affected and it becomes swollen, red, hot, and very painful. Other possible causes of mastitis are fatigue, stress, a tight-fitting bra, infrequent changing of wet nursing pads, or a sudden change in the baby's nursing pattern. Occasionally, bacteria will enter the breast through an opening in the nipple or a break in the skin and cause mastitis. Mastitis is most common during the early days of nursing and when a mother is not getting the proper rest and nutrition she needs. Identifying and treating mastitis immediately could mean the difference between a few hours of discomfort or several days in bed.

Treating Mastitis:

- Contact your doctor as soon as you notice symptoms. Mastitis is usually treated with antibiotics that can be taken while nursing. If symptoms continue after 3 days of treatment, contact your doctor. (A delay in treating mastitis could lead to a *breast abscess*, a localized infection that may need to be treated surgically).
- Rest is necessary at the first sign of a problem. Relax and lie down as much as possible. Get help with all other chores.
- Continue nursing often around the clock. Nursing keeps the milk flowing and the infection from becoming worse. Your milk is safe for your baby because of the antibacterial properties of breast milk.
- Apply warm, moist compresses on the sore area before and during a nursing session (such as a warm, moist washcloth). You may also try soaking your breast by leaning over a basin of warm water for several minutes.
- Nurse on the unaffected breast first to lessen discomfort. Nursing on the affected breast may be somewhat painful, but should not be avoided.
- If your baby does not empty the affected breast as completely as possible, hand express or pump the milk that is left.
- While you recover, don't wear a bra, if it is more comfortable.
- Make sure you are eating a nutritious diet and drinking plenty of fluids.
- Talk to your doctor about a pain reliever approved for breastfeeding mothers.
- If the mastitis returns, talk to your doctor to determine the cause.

Thrush

If your nipple area becomes pink, flaky, or itchy and your nipples are cracked, red, or burning, you may have *thrush.* Thrush is a yeast infection caused by an overgrowth of the fungus *Candida albicans.* *Candida albicans* is found naturally in our bodies and grows in warm, dark places and thrives on milk. Thrush isn't serious, but it can be painful and it may hurt to nurse. If your baby has it in his mouth, you may see white patches on his tongue and inside his cheeks. It is usually spread from the baby's mouth to the mother's nipples. Thrush may also cause your baby to have a bright red diaper rash, and you may have a vaginal yeast infection. Yet, sometimes a baby with thrush may have no symptoms at all. Since *Candida* is found in the birth canal, thrush can also be passed to the baby during a vaginal birth. Or, it can be caused by antibiotics given to the mother or the baby. Thrush is more prone to develop in women with diabetes. If you or your baby are having symptoms of thrush, contact your doctor for treatment. You must treat thrush as soon as you notice symptoms to prevent reinfection, but there is no need to stop nursing.

Preventing Thrush:

- Wash your hands thoroughly before each feeding and after each diaper change.
- Change nursing pads and diapers often. Avoid nursing pads with plastic liners because they prevent air circulation.
- Avoid using nipple creams or lotions, which may help the growth of yeast-like fungus or bacteria.
- Eat yogurt with active cultures to help keep the yeast organisms in check.

Treating Thrush:

- Contact your baby's doctor (and if necessary, your own doctor) for medication, which is usually Nystatin (mycostatin) ointment or drops. To prevent reinfection, it is necessary to treat both you and your baby at the same time.
- Wash your hands before each feeding and after each diaper change.
- Rinse your breasts with plain warm water after each feeding and apply the medication as prescribed.
- Rinse your baby's mouth with plain water after each feeding and apply the medication as prescribed. Medication for your baby's diaper area may also be prescribed if he has a rash.
- Change nursing pads and diapers often. Avoid nursing pads with plastic liners because they prevent air circulation.
- During a bout of thrush, any expressed breast milk should be used immediately or thrown away to prevent reinfection. (Do not freeze breast milk that was pumped during the infection for later use. Yeast is not destroyed by freezing.)
- Wash all breast pump parts thoroughly after each use. Boil any breast-pump parts that come into contact with your breast milk each day.
- Thoroughly wash and boil anything that goes into your baby's mouth (rubber nipples, pacifiers, teethers, toys, etc.).
- Wash bras in hot, soapy water each day and rinse well.
- If thrush seems to be persistent, you may also need to treat your partner, since thrush can be easily transmitted through intimate contact.

Low Milk Supply

Almost all new mothers are able to produce enough milk for their babies if they breastfeed often and long enough. Only a very small percentage of women are unable to produce enough breast milk for their infants. Consult your doctor or a lactation specialist if you feel your milk supply is low, or your baby does not regain his birth weight by 2 weeks of age. The following tips will help you increase your milk supply.

Ways to Increase Your Milk Supply:

- Nurse often, at least every 2 to 3 hours around the clock.
- Encourage your baby to nurse as often and as long as he wishes.
- Wake your baby to nurse, if necessary.
- Make sure your baby is positioned correctly at your breast during each feeding.
- Offer both breasts. Encourage your baby to empty both breasts as completely as possible at each feeding. (You may need to pump the milk that is left.)
- Try "switch nursing": nurse on one breast until your baby begins to lose interest, burp him, then switch breasts. Repeat 2 to 3 times during each feeding.
- Feed your baby *only* breast milk. Do not supplement with formula or water.
- Avoid using bottles and pacifiers. All sucking should be done at the breast.
- Make sure you are comfortable and relaxed during feedings. Tension may slow down your milk flow.
- Try to get enough rest and sleep when your baby sleeps, or at least lie down to nurse.
- Drink plenty of fluids and eat a nutritious diet.
- Pumping may give your breasts additional stimulation and increase your milk supply. After each feeding, use a pump for at least 10 minutes on each breast to empty them as completely as possible. A high-grade electric breast pump is most effective for increasing your milk supply.

Breastfeeding 911: Getting Help

Recognizing False Alarms

There may be times when you will wonder if you are making enough milk for your baby because of your baby's behavior or symptoms you may be having. Most of the time, they are just false alarms and nothing to worry about. As long as your baby looks healthy, is nursing often, gaining weight, and having enough wet and soiled diapers, your milk supply is probably fine. There is usually no need to worry about any of the following:

- *Your breasts suddenly don't seem as full as they were before.* As your milk production adjusts to your baby's needs, and the early engorgement passes, your breasts may not seem as full. This is normal.
- *Your breasts no longer leak.* Leaking doesn't have anything to do with your milk production. Leaking may become less of a problem once your milk supply is matched to your baby's needs.
- *You don't feel the let-down reflex, or the feeling isn't as strong as it was before.* Some mothers never feel the let-down reflex and for others it becomes less noticeable over time.
- *Your baby nurses very often but still seems hungry soon after being nursed.* Remember that breast milk is quickly and easily digested, and babies nurse for comfort as well as food. Your baby may also be going through a growth spurt. This is when your baby nurses more often than usual to increase your milk supply to meet his growing needs. Growth spurts occur at about 2 weeks, 6 weeks, 3 months, and 6 months of age. Your baby will soon settle back into a less demanding nursing pattern.

- *Your baby nurses less often and nurses for shorter periods.* Babies become better and better at getting milk from the breast over time. Nursing sessions may gradually shorten or your baby may nurse less often.
- *Your baby is fussy.* Most babies have normal fussy periods. There are many reasons for a baby to fuss besides hunger. If nursing doesn't help, try a walk, a warm bath, a massage, rocking him, or swaddling him in a blanket. But if fussiness is constant, or your baby has other symptoms, it may be a sign of a medical problem. Call your baby's doctor.
- *Your baby's weight gain, nursing patterns, and general routines are different from other babies you know.* Each child is unique and has his own routines and growth pattern. There are wide variations within the normal range of healthy babies. However, if you strongly feel something is wrong with your baby, talk to your baby's doctor.

Who to Call for Help

The following section will help you decide whether to call a lactation specialist or the doctor, depending on the problem you are having.

When to Call the Lactation Specialist

You should quickly get the help of a lactation specialist if you are experiencing any of the following:

- You are unable to position your baby for nursing.
- Your baby has not nursed during the first 12 hours after birth.
- After the first day of life, your baby nurses fewer than 8 times in a 24-hour period or cannot be awakened to nurse at least every 3 hours.
- Your baby seems hungry but nurses at your breast for only a minute or two.
- Your breasts continue to be engorged at the end of a feeding.
- Your nipples are painful, cracked, blistered, or bleeding.
- You are tempted to supplement feedings with formula because you are afraid you don't have enough breast milk.
- Your baby's weight gain is poor (fewer than 4 ounces per week, counting from your baby's lowest weight, not from his birth weight).

When to Call the Doctor

Call the doctor if either you or your baby have any of the following warning signs:

Warning Signs for Mother (call your doctor):

- You have very heavy bright red bleeding after the 3rd day and are soaking more than one sanitary pad per hour, or are passing large blood clots. (See "Physical Changes" on PAGE 65.)
- You have a fever higher than 100°F.
- You have swelling, a foul odor, or discharge from the episiotomy area.
- Your cesarean incision is opened, has a foul odor, is red, or has a discharge.
- You have an area on your breast that is hot, hard, red, and painful to touch. (See "Mastitis" on PAGE 55.)

- You have severe abdominal pain.
- You have a burning sensation when you urinate.
- You have a persistent headache, dizziness, or are seeing spots.
- You have swelling of the face, feet, or fingers.
- You have an area in your calf or leg that is red, swollen, hard, and painful.
- You have postpartum depression for longer than 2 weeks. (See "Emotional Changes" on PAGE 66.)

Warning Signs for Baby (call your baby's doctor):

- Your baby will not nurse and has missed 2 or more feedings in a row.
- Your baby's stools are still black after the 4th day. (See "Meconium" on PAGE 30.)
- Your baby has fewer than 2 stools per day after the 4th day.
- Your baby has fewer than 6 wet diapers per day after the 4th day.
- Your baby's stools have blood, mucus, or a foul odor; or they are very loose or watery. (See "Diarrhea" on PAGE 47.)
- Your baby always seems hungry after a feeding.
- Your baby is unusually irritable, very sleepy, restless, or lethargic.
- Your baby is very difficult to wake.
- Your baby has difficulty breathing, flaring nostrils, or wheezing congestion.
- Your baby has a fever higher than 100°F (rectal temperature).
- Your baby's umbilical cord is swollen, red, or foul-smelling; or there is drainage, excessive bleeding, or redness of the surrounding skin.
- Your baby vomits frequently, excessively, and forcefully or vomits a bright-green bile liquid. (See "Vomiting" on PAGE 47.)
- Your baby's skin is hot, moist, perspiring, or blotchy.
- Your baby's skin and the whites of his eyes have a yellow color. (See "Jaundice" on PAGE 46.)
- Your baby has excessive tearing, swelling, redness, or discharge from his eyes.
- Your baby has white patches on his tongue and inside his cheeks. (See "Thrush" on PAGE 55.)
- Your baby's belly feels swollen and hard and he has been constipated for more than 24 hours. (See "Constipation" on PAGE 48.)
- Your baby shows signs of dehydration. (See "Signs of Dehydration" on PAGE 35.)
- You feel something is wrong with your baby, but you are not sure what it is.

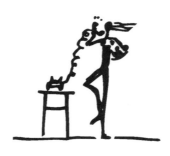

Getting Over the Six-Week Hurdle

The first 6 weeks after birth can be a difficult time for many new mothers. If they are having difficulties, some new mothers just don't believe that breastfeeding will get any easier. Unfortunately, many babies are weaned between 4 and 6 weeks of age. Most of the time, it is because the mother feels she is not making enough breast milk for her baby. But this is usually not what is happening. Mothers sometimes lose their confidence around this time because their babies seem to be fussier than before, and this behavior is automatically blamed on a low milk supply. But you must realize that a 4- to 6-week old baby is sometimes a rather fussy little person. He is becoming more aware of his surroundings and is more sensitive to noises, lights, darkness, and dirty diapers. He is beginning to know the feeling of loneliness when you are not around. He is trying to get used to his new, unfamiliar world—so he cries and fusses more. At 6 weeks, your baby may seem to want to nurse "all the time," because he is probably going through a growth spurt.

Some mothers who stop breastfeeding around this time decide that they just don't want to be a human bottle anymore—always nursing their child. They decide that breastfeeding takes too much time and effort and they can't imagine continuing at this pace. They feel as if they will never again have enough time to take a shower, clean their house, have a social life, or a peaceful night's sleep. Although these new mothers can physically do more, their bodies are still recovering from childbirth, so they become overly tired trying to get things done.

This is the time you may think of weaning your baby. But giving your baby a bottle of formula won't make your baby's needs go away. In fact, making the change from breast milk to formula may take much more of your time and energy than you think. Remember, if you switch to formula you will have to wash and sterilize bottles and nipples and prepare and warm it. And you still have to take time out to hold your baby while feeding him a bottle of formula. It may also take several days before your baby adjusts to this new liquid being put into his body, since his digestive system is already used to breast milk. In some cases, giving a baby cow's milk formula may cause an allergic reaction or digestive problems such as gas, diarrhea, or constipation—and along with stomach upset comes more fussiness and crying. Even if your baby takes the formula and goes longer between feedings, the little time you gain is not worth giving up the lifetime benefits of breastfeeding.

The 6-week learning period is the most difficult phase of breastfeeding. But it is the turning point—and not the time to give up! Breastfeeding your baby does become easier after this period. A few weeks from now you will look back on these days and wonder why you ever doubted yourself. In most cases, beginning about the seventh week, things begin to change and breastfeeding your baby becomes much easier. Your baby is no longer the fragile newborn you brought home from the hospital, whose only waking interest was breastfeeding. As your baby grows, his digestive system matures. He becomes better at breastfeeding and goes longer between feedings and has longer stretches of sleep at night. Nursing your baby starts to become easier. Problems such as nipple soreness, engorgement, and leaking have worked themselves out. Your body has become used to the breastfeeding process. Your baby is becoming more interested in his surroundings. He is now starting to respond to you. He smiles, looks at you lovingly, and is starting to become sociable. He is happier because you are able to read his signs more easily, which makes him much easier to care for than when he was a newborn. You are able to get more things done. You are feeling more like yourself and much more relaxed and confident in caring for your baby. Outings become much easier, with or without your baby, and you look forward to nights out with your partner again. You enjoy your baby's company, and a loving relationship between mother and child is growing. You finally understand the sparkle in the eyes of nursing mothers when they talk about the beauty of breastfeeding a baby. You have come to appreciate the joy of breastfeeding!

If You Are Not Able to Continue Breastfeeding

If, for whatever reason, you are not able to continue breastfeeding your baby, hold your head up high and be proud of yourself for trying. You have done your best to give your baby the best. Your love for your baby can still show when you bottle-feed him with formula. You can bottle-feed your baby like a breastfeeding mother by giving him close skin-to-skin contact and your full attention throughout the feeding. Change your baby from side to side to help develop better hand-eye coordination. Wear your baby in a sling for added closeness and you can even keep your baby in your room or bed at night. Know that you have done your best under your circumstances, and that breastfeeding for whatever amount of time has made a difference.

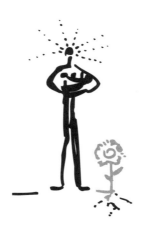

CHAPTER 4

Special Situations

Breastfeeding After a Cesarean

Even if you have had a cesarean delivery, your body will still be able to make milk for your baby. Just as in a vaginal delivery, the normal hormonal process that starts milk production begins as soon as your baby is born. If your cesarean delivery is planned, you can prepare ahead of time by letting your doctor know you want to breastfeed. Once you are at the hospital you can remind the hospital staff before the surgery that you want to breastfeed early and often. If you have an unplanned cesarean delivery, you can still breastfeed, even if medical complications don't allow you to nurse immediately after the birth. If you had general anesthesia, you may feel a little drowsy. As soon as you are feeling more alert, and as long as you and your baby are both doing well, try to have your baby with you in your room as much as possible. Breastfeeding often in the hospital will bring you and your baby emotionally and physically close, and give you a sense of confidence knowing that you can nourish your baby. If you or your baby need special care and will not be able to start breastfeeding for more than 24 to 48 hours, you may need to work with a lactation specialist to pump your breast milk.

After a cesarean delivery, you may be given pain medication for several days that is safe for both you and your baby. Because you are recovering from surgery, it might be difficult to find a comfortable position to nurse. You may have to ask for help from the nursing staff or your partner. It is important to find a position that will not harm your incision or be uncomfortable. While your incision is healing, the side-lying position works well. If you prefer to sit up, the football hold position keeps the baby's weight off your abdomen. Breastfeeding after a cesarean delivery may be a bit more difficult in the beginning, since the healing process takes a little longer than for a normal vaginal delivery—but nursing your baby will be just as rewarding.

Breastfeeding the Premature Baby

If your baby is born prematurely, it is especially important that he receive breast milk. Some premature babies may weigh less than 2 pounds when they are born and need to be kept in an *isolette* (a small incubator) in the hospital for a month or longer. These babies may be fed breast milk through a tube and may not be ready to nurse at the breast for several weeks. Other babies who weigh closer to 5 pounds may be able to nurse soon after birth. Whatever your situation, breast milk is even more valuable to your premature baby. When you deliver prematurely, your body produces milk that is different from regular breast milk and helps your baby grow faster, stronger, and healthier. This milk is higher in calories and important nutrients, including protein, fat, and sodium, to meet your premature baby's special needs. It also has greater amounts of antibodies that are so important for your premature baby's health. Breast milk is also more easily digested and causes less stress on your tiny baby's system. If your premature baby is unable to breastfeed, you will need to pump your breasts and feed him your expressed breast milk. This also keeps your milk flowing until your baby is ready to nurse. Your premature baby should eat at least every 3 hours around the clock or whenever he shows signs of hunger.

When your premature baby is ready to nurse at the breast, breastfeeding is the best way to make up for the time the two of you were separated. But keep in mind that learning to latch on can be especially difficult for premature babies. Most babies don't develop the suck-swallow-breathe reflex that is necessary for nursing until about 32 weeks in the womb. But with a little patience, determination, and the proper help, your baby will be breastfeeding as soon as he is ready. For more help, talk to a lactation specialist or contact La Leche League about breastfeeding premature babies. They can guide you and put you in touch with other mothers who have successfully nursed premature babies.

Breastfeeding Multiples

Breastfeeding multiples may be a little more challenging—but the rewards will be multiplied! Thousands of mothers have successfully nursed two or more babies. Since multiples are often born early, your breast milk will be especially important to them. Breastfeeding is also a perfect way to develop a special relationship with each of your babies. Because the law of "supply and demand" also works for mothers of multiples, your body is able to make enough milk to meet the nutritional needs of two or more infants. With multiples, you can choose to breastfeed exclusively or you can supplement breastfeeding with formula, depending on your needs and your particular situation. Whichever method you choose, remember that any amount of breastfeeding will greatly benefit your babies.

Things can get hectic with two or more babies, but it is important to make sure that each baby gets 8 to 12 feedings every 24 hours. This may mean keeping careful track of your babies' feeding times and wet and soiled diapers for the first few weeks. If one or more of the babies are born prematurely, you will need to begin pumping as soon as possible after birth at the same times your baby (or babies) would nurse, at least every 2 to 3 hours. If you are breastfeeding or pumping frequently, you can trust that your body will make enough milk for your babies. A low milk supply can usually be corrected by nursing or pumping more often. You can either nurse one baby at a time or two babies at the same time. The football hold works well for nursing two babies at the same time; however, there are other positions you may find more comfortable. You will eventually find one that works best for all of you. Try to get as much help as you can from the nurses or a lactation specialist before you leave the hospital. For more help with breastfeeding multiples, contact an organization that has support groups for parents of multiples such as La Leche League or Mothers of Twins.

CHAPTER 5

Adjusting to Motherhood

Childbirth is a dramatic, life-changing event and getting used to your new role as mother may take some time. You will be going through many changes during the first few weeks postpartum, both physically and emotionally. After the delivery, it is important to remember the birth experience and ease yourself into your new role as mother. Knowing what to expect during these early days can help make adjusting to your new life a little easier.

During the first 6 weeks postpartum you will be recovering from the physical stress of pregnancy and labor and the highly emotional experience of childbirth. As your life changes, it is natural to feel many different emotions—from excitement and joy to worry and disappointment. Your new role as mother may not be exactly what you thought. Caring for your newborn may take a lot more time and energy than you ever imagined. Your baby's many needs may seem endless. You may feel that you will never again have a good night's sleep. Breastfeeding may not be as easy as you expected. You may feel unsure of yourself and question your own mothering skills. Motherhood may not seem at all like the pictures in the parenting magazines. But don't worry—with so many changes happening in the early days, it is normal to have mixed feelings about breastfeeding and motherhood. Just remember that they both get easier with time. Soon you will settle into your new life. The most important thing you can do during this time is to take good care of yourself. The better you take care of yourself, the better you will be able to take care of your baby—and soon you will feel confident in your new role as mother.

During difficult times of mothering, it helps to look at things a little differently by putting yourself in your "baby's booties." Think about what *he* has just been through and imagine how *he* must feel—then follow the "golden rule" and treat him the way you would want to be treated. Remind yourself how lucky you are to have this new little person in your life and how much richer and more meaningful your days will be. Think of all the wonderful times you are going to share with this new love of your life. And for now, you are the center of his world, and as far as he is concerned, you are perfect!

Physical Changes

Immediately after the birth, as your uterus returns to its normal size, you will have a vaginal discharge called **lochia**. This is the shedding of the uterine lining and is similar to a heavy menstrual period. This discharge will be bright red for approximately 1 to 3 days. Over the next 2 weeks the flow will gradually become medium to light as the color changes from bright red to watery pink, then to brown, and finally to yellowish-white or colorless. Breastfeeding helps the uterus shrink back to its normal size more quickly and reduces the flow of lochia by causing uterine contractions and constricting uterine blood vessels.

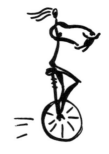

As your uterus gradually shrinks and makes its way back into the pelvis, you may feel mild contractions known as *after-pains*. These **after-pains** feel similar to menstrual cramps and may be mild to fairly strong. During the first few days postpartum, they may become stronger when you are nursing your baby, since *oxytocin*, the same hormone that delivers milk to your baby, also causes your uterus to contract. These after-pains should lessen within a few days.

If you had an **episiotomy**, which is an incision to enlarge the vaginal opening, or a tear in the vaginal area, it may feel painful and sensitive. After the birth, an ice pack will numb the pain and reduce the swelling. Later, a cool sitz bath (a shallow bath filled with water) may bring relief. Sometimes alternating heat and cold may also be helpful. Keep the area clean and dry, and wear cotton underwear. Episiotomy pain usually improves daily with proper care, and the stitches should dissolve in about two weeks.

While your body is adjusting from a pregnant to a non-pregnant state, you will also be going through enormous hormonal changes. These hormonal ups and downs can have a strong effect on your mood and may cause you to feel a variety of unexpected emotions.

Emotional Changes

After the birth of your baby you may have a wide range of emotions—including some unexpected highs and lows. No matter how much you looked forward to your baby's arrival, after the high feeling that comes with childbirth you may have a temporary low period. The waiting and planning that have been a big part of your life for the last several months have come to end. The focus of everyone's attention has changed from the expectant mother to the precious new baby. This emotional letdown is partly due to the hormonal changes going on in your body. Additionally, your body is in the process of returning to its non-pregnant state and your milk-producing hormones are working overtime to bring in your milk supply. And to top it off, you are now suddenly responsible for being the full-time caregiver of a new baby who is totally dependent upon you. It's no wonder you are on such an emotional roller coaster!

This very common condition is called the *baby blues* and may suddenly appear on the third or fourth day after the delivery. You may also find yourself crying for no reason. Other symptoms of the **baby blues** may include irritability, anxiety, impatience, fatigue, and restlessness. These feelings are usually due to a combination of the following four things: (1) the emotional letdown after giving birth, (2) the hormonal changes in your body, (3) a sudden awareness of your new responsibilities, and (4) exhaustion due to the lack of sleep. You may have a few difficult days, but within a week or two things should improve. During this period, love and support from your partner, family, and friends are very important. Ask for their emotional support, share your feelings with them, and accept their help. It also helps to share your feelings with other new mothers who know how you feel. Exercise (with your doctor's approval) is another way to improve your mood and will help you lose postpartum pounds. Getting outdoors and walking with your baby is the perfect exercise during these early weeks. But the best cure for the baby blues is time. Symptoms usually improve within 1 to 2 weeks as your hormone levels return to normal and you become more confident in caring for your baby.

For some new mothers the baby blues may turn into *postpartum depression* which can occur within days of the delivery or appear slowly over the next several months. You may have **postpartum depression** if you have any of the following symptoms: anxiety, mental confusion, despair, insomnia, intense worry, or panic. A new mother with postpartum depression may cry uncontrollably, be withdrawn, have a change in eating habits (loss of appetite or overeating), and may express irrational fears about herself and her baby. The exact cause of postpartum depression is unclear, but women who suffer from postpartum depression are more likely to have been depressed in the past or have a family history of mood disorders.

A new mother struggling with postpartum depression may find nursing to be difficult, since getting a good amount of sleep is very important in helping those who are suffering from any type of mood disorder. If you are suffering from postpartum depression and don't want to give up your breastfeeding relationship with your baby, one way to help you get at least 5 to 6 hours of sleep at night is to pump your breast milk during the day and have your partner handle the nighttime feedings. However, if breastfeeding becomes too overwhelming, know that the time you did spend breastfeeding was beneficial to both you and your baby.

In all cases of postpartum depression, getting proper help is an important step toward recovery. Treatment for postpartum depression may include counseling or in some cases antidepressant medication. (There are certain antidepressant medications that are currently thought to be safe for breastfeeding mothers.) If you are experiencing any of the symptoms of postpartum depression or you are having thoughts of harming yourself or your baby, contact your doctor for appropriate treatment.

Relationship Changes

Motherhood not only changes your life, but it also changes your relationships with those close to you—in one way or another. Having a child helps you see things through different eyes. It helps you take another look at your own life and adds a new layer to all other relationships.

When partners become parents it's easy to lose touch with each other, which may create conflict and separation. Caring for a newborn takes so much time and energy that there is little time left to focus on anything else—including your relationship with your partner. Some days you may feel like your partner is not doing enough. You may feel jealous of his freedom as he leaves for the day. On the other hand, your partner may be jealous of your close relationship with your baby, and he may feel left out of the family circle. There may be days when you both look at your baby and then look at each other and wonder "What have we done?" These feelings and reactions are normal when partners become parents. However, it is important to understand what is happening and take time out to reconnect. Try to communicate your feelings and your needs to each other as much as possible. As difficult as it may seem, try to spend time alone together and get to know each other again. Talk about the day you met and the qualities that brought you together as a couple. Discuss how these qualities will help you in raising your child. Realize that parenting is a team effort and in order for your child to feel a sense of family togetherness, there needs to be love and harmony in your relationship with your partner. Soon the day will come when your child does something wonderful and you will look at each other and say "Look what we've done!"

After having a child, the word "family" takes on a whole new meaning. Not only are you a member of a family, you are now the creator of one. Your close family ties may become stronger as you gain a new understanding and appreciation of your own parents and siblings. You may especially feel a new respect for your own mother. Family members will play an important and influential role in your child's life. Each of these relationships will be unique and will enrich your child's life in different ways. Watching these relationships develop and grow will bring your own relationship with each family member to a new level.

Because having a child is one of the most courageous things a woman can do, it creates a strong connection to all mothers. As a new mother, you may feel the joy and pain of other mothers more deeply than ever before. You may also have very strong feelings for another child's tears and feel light-hearted when you hear the sound of another child's laughter. These powerful feelings are the universal bond of motherhood at work.

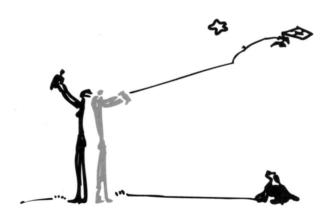

CHAPTER 6

Nutrition For the Nursing Mother

Breastfeeding Nutrition

As a new mother, eating a healthy diet will make you feel good and help you recover from childbirth. It will also give you the energy you need to take care of your new baby—because with a new baby in the house, you need all the energy you can get! Some mothers think that if they eat a poor diet—for example skipping meals or choosing unhealthy foods—their breast milk will not be good. But even mothers who don't always eat well still have good breast milk. This is because a nursing mother's body is amazingly able to store and use any nutrients the mother takes in to create nutritious breast milk. A mother's diet would have to be very poor for a long period of time for her milk to be lacking nutrients. However, if you are not eating well, the nutrients needed to keep up the quality of your breast milk will come from your own body's nutrient stores. This may cause you to feel tired and weak and could eventually slow down your milk production.

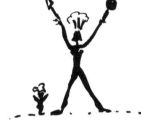

Many mothers think that if they breastfeed, they have to eat a special diet. But, the good news is, you don't have to stop eating the foods you love in order to breastfeed! The goal of this chapter is to show you how to take the foods you normally eat and turn them into a balanced diet by using the *USDA Food Guide Pyramid* and the *U.S. Food Exchange System*. These eating guides divide foods into separate categories or "food groups" according to their nutritional content. All the foods we eat every day fit into one or more of these food groups. Because every food has a place in our diets, no food is off limits! Of course, some foods are healthier than others and in order to balance your diet there are certain food groups you should eat from more often than others—but all foods are allowed.

Even while breastfeeding, your baby is becoming familiar with and learning to like the foods you eat through your breast milk. After your child is no longer breastfeeding, he will learn what to eat by watching you, so now is a perfect time to make sure you are eating a healthy diet. To get you started and help you stay on track, you can use the **"Nursing Mother's Daily Nutrition Checklist"** beginning on PAGE 84. This one-week food diary will guide you on your way to healthy eating by helping you put into action what you learn in this chapter.

Breastfeeding and Weight Loss

Breastfeeding makes it easier for new mothers to lose their pregnancy weight because making breast milk can burn from 500 to 800 calories per day! These extra calories will come from the fat stores you gained during pregnancy and the food you eat. By eating a balanced diet at a calorie level that is right for you, you can naturally lose your pregnancy weight over a period of 4 to 6 months.

Most new mothers expect to lose a large amount of weight immediately after the delivery, but the amount of weight loss from childbirth varies from woman to woman. Some women find that they temporarily hold on to extra fluid, and the weight loss doesn't show up on the scale until several days after the delivery, as their bodies gradually get rid of this extra fluid. Also, while you are nursing, your breasts may weigh more by a pound or two. Generally, you may naturally lose from 10 to 20 pounds from childbirth during the first 2 to 3 weeks after the delivery. After that, if you are breastfeeding exclusively, eating at the right calorie level, and making wise food choices, you can expect to lose from 1 to 2 pounds per week. Just remember to take it slowly, and don't expect to lose weight too quickly. Respect your body, feed it with nutritious foods, and give it proper rest—and it will happily take care of you and your baby!

Daily Calorie Requirement

It is recommended that nursing mothers eat an extra 200 to 500 calories per day to support milk production. For most nursing mothers, that means eating between 1,800 and 2,200 calories per day. The number of calories you need depends on your size, your activity level, and the amount of breast milk you are making. For example, a mother who is breastfeeding *exclusively* will need more calories than a mother who is nursing *and* giving her baby formula. You will naturally feel hungrier and thirstier while breastfeeding, so satisfying your hunger and thirst should usually bring you up to your daily calorie level. Most women can start with a calorie intake of 1,800 calories per day. However, if you are tall or exercise regularly, you may want to start with 2,200 calories per day. The best way to tell if you are eating the right number of calories is to weigh yourself and listen to your body. If you are losing weight too quickly or your energy level is low, you may need to increase your calorie intake. If you are gaining weight, you may need to lower your calorie intake. Just make sure to eat at least 1,800 calories each day to ensure that you have a good milk supply without tapping into your own body's nutrient stores. Going below 1,800 calories per day makes it difficult to get all the nutrients you need to breastfeed successfully. If you are very underweight or overweight, are nursing multiples, or have special dietary needs, talk to a nutritionist for dietary recommendations.

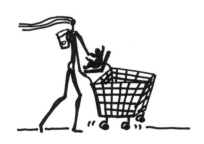

The USDA Food Guide Pyramid

The **USDA Food Guide Pyramid** gives you a visual image of how to plan a healthy diet. It puts foods that are similar in nutrients into "food groups" and suggests how many servings from each group you should have each day. The base of the pyramid shows you that grains form the foundation of a healthy diet. Next are vegetables and fruits, and then milk and meat. Fats, oils, and sweets are represented by only a tiny triangle at the top of the pyramid because they provide very few nutrients and should be eaten in moderation.

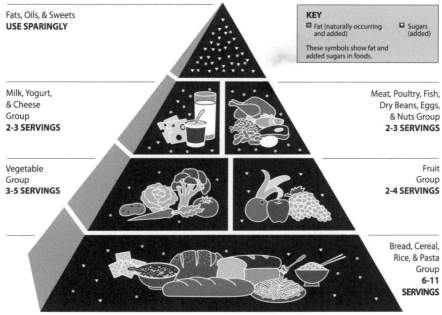

Source: U.S. Department of Agriculture/U.S. Department of Health and Human Services

The U.S. Food Exchange System

The **U.S. Food Exchange System** is another diet planning tool that groups foods a little differently. It puts foods that are similar in *carbohydrates*, *protein*, and *fat* (energy nutrients) into different "exchange lists." Each food serving on a given list has approximately the same amount of carbohydrates, protein, and fat, and the same number of calories as any other food serving on that same list. So the foods on a list can be exchanged, or traded, for each other without affecting the plan's balance or total calories. This meal planning system helps people with diabetes but can be a useful tool for anyone by making it easier to watch your calorie and fat intake and balance your diet. According to the **Dietary Guidelines for Americans,** a balanced diet includes:

- 55–60% calories from carbohydrates
- 15–20% calories from protein
- 30% or less calories from fat

Your Daily Food Group Servings

Using the food group plan together with the exchange lists can make it easier to plan a healthy diet. Putting foods into "food groups" allows you to choose a certain number of servings from each group and offers variety. The exchange lists ensure that the foods in each group are equal in energy nutrients and calories and offer balance. Following the guidelines of the USDA Food Guide Pyramid and the U.S. Food Exchange System, the table below breaks down foods into 6 different food groups—grains, vegetables, fruits, dairy, protein, and fats—and shows you the recommended number of servings from each group for nursing mothers at five different calorie levels.

Daily Food Group Servings for Nursing Mothers						
Calories	Grains	Vegetables	Fruits	Dairy	Protein	Fats
1,800	7	4	4	3	4	4
2,000	8	4	4	3	4	5
2,200	9	4	4	4	4	6
2,400	11	4	4	4	4	7
2,600	12	4	4	4	4	8

Choose the calorie level that is right for you and fill in the table below with the correct number of food group servings.

My Personal Food Group Servings						
Calories	Grains	Vegetables	Fruits	Dairy	Protein	Fats

Food Exchange Lists

This section shows you the food exchange lists for the 6 different food groups: grains, vegetables, fruits, dairy, protein, and fats. Use the exchange lists to help you plan a healthy diet and to record your food intake in the "Nursing Mother's Daily Nutrition Checklist" beginning on PAGE 84. After each list, it explains why that food group is important and gives you tips on how to get enough in your diet. Suggested number of servings, calories per serving, and serving sizes are also included with each list.

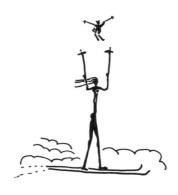

Grains
(Bread, Cereal, Rice, Pasta & Starchy Vegetables)

- 7–12 servings per day
- Approximately 80 calories per serving
- Amounts listed are one serving size

Beans, peas, lentils, corn, cooked (½ cup)	Pasta, whole-grain, white, cooked (½ cup)
Bread, whole-grain, white, sliced (1)	Popcorn, popped, fat-free (3 cups)
Bread sticks, 4-inch (2)	Potato, baked (1 small)
Bun, hot dog, hamburger (½)	Potato, mashed (½ cup)
Cereal, fortified, cold (¾ cup)	Rice, risotto, cooked (⅓ cup)
Cereal, fortified, hot (½ cup)	Rice cakes (2)
Couscous, polenta, cooked (⅓ cup)	Squash, pumpkin (1 cup)
Crackers, pretzels (¾ oz.)	Sweet potato, yam (½ cup)
Dinner roll (1)	Tortilla, pita, 6-inch (1)
English muffin, bagel (½)	Waffle, pancake, low-fat (1)
Graham crackers (3 squares)	Wheat germ (3 tbs.)

Grain products and **starchy vegetables** provide you with **carbohydrates** (or carbs), your body's main source of energy. They also provide B vitamins to help your body use the energy and iron for healthy blood. There are two types of carbohydrates: *simple carbohydrates* and *complex carbohydrates*.

Simple carbohydrates are grain products made from refined flours and sugars such as cookies, cakes, doughnuts, pastries, and sugary cereals. These foods are made of simple sugars that are absorbed quickly into your bloodstream and cause a sudden rise and fall in blood sugar, which creates a craving for more. Eating these foods too often can also contribute to adult-onset diabetes. These foods should play only a small part in your diet.

Complex carbohydrates such as whole-grain breads and cereals and starchy vegetables are your best choices since they are the highest in nutrients and fiber and lowest in fat. Complex carbohydrates enter the bloodstream more slowly and do not cause a sudden rise and fall in blood sugar. They also take longer for your body to digest so they keep you satisfied longer.

TIPS:

- You can find whole-grain versions of most grain products (whole-gain breads, whole-grain cereals, whole-grain pastas, whole-grain tortillas, and brown rice) in your local grocery store.
- Try to eat at least 3 whole-grain foods each day. (The fiber will help with postpartum constipation.)
- Try different types of whole-grain breads and grain-based dishes such as couscous, risotto, or polenta.

Vegetables

- **4 servings per day**
- **Approximately 25 calories per serving**
- **Eat at least one vegetable (or fruit), high in vitamin A each day**
- **One serving size is: 1 cup raw, ½ cup cooked, or ½ cup juice**

Artichokes	Brussels sprouts	Eggplant	Mustard greens	Spinach
Asparagus	Cabbage	Green beans	Okra	Tomatoes
Bean sprouts	Carrots	Jicama	Onions	Turnip greens
Beets	Cauliflower	Kale	Peppers	Turnips
Bok choy	Celery	Leeks	Radishes	Water chestnuts
Broccoli	Cucumber	Mushrooms	Snow peas	Zucchini

Vegetables are another source of **complex carbohydrates** and are rich in vitamin A and folic acid as well as vitamin C and fiber. **Vitamin A** helps keep your eyes and skin healthy and reduces the risk of infections and certain cancers. **It is important to eat at least one vegetable (or fruit) high in vitamin A each day. Some foods high in vitamin A include kale, turnip greens, spinach, carrots, sweet potatoes, red bell peppers, tomatoes, broccoli, mangos, apricots, and cantaloupe. Folic acid** (folate) is a B vitamin that helps our bodies make new cells. Getting enough folic acid in your diet is important, especially if you are planning another pregnancy, as it can help prevent major birth defects of a baby's brain and spine known as *neural tube defects* or *NTDs*. Women need to eat foods high in folic acid every day *before* they become pregnant to help prevent NTDs. **Foods that contain folic acid include dark green leafy vegetables, asparagus, spinach, Brussels sprouts, broccoli, legumes, wheat germ, eggs, orange juice, fortified cereals, and enriched grain products.**

TIPS:

- Enjoy the vegetables you have always eaten—just eat more of them.
- For more fiber, keep edible peels on vegetables such as cucumbers and zucchini.
- Add grated or shredded vegetables such as zucchini or carrots to lasagna, meat loaf, mashed potatoes, and pasta dishes.
- Try something new such as Brussels sprouts, kale, turnip greens, leeks, or bok choy.
- Chop and wash vegetables all at one time and store them in plastic bags in the refrigerator for snacking.

Fruits

- **4 servings per day**
- **Approximately 60 calories per serving**
- **Eat at least one fruit (or vegetable) high in vitamin C each day**
- **Amounts listed are one serving size**

Apple (1 medium)	Dried fruit (¼ cup)	Mango (½ medium)	Pear (1 medium)
Apricots (4 small)	Fruit juice (½ cup)	Melon (1 cup)	Pineapple (1 cup)
Banana (1 medium)	Fruit nectar (¼ cup)	Nectarine (2 small)	Plums (2 small)
Berries, all types (1 cup)	Grapefruit (½ medium)	Orange (1 medium)	Tangerines (2 small)
Cantaloupe (1 cup)	Grapes (12 large)	Papaya (½ medium)	
Cherries (12 large)	Kiwi (1 medium)	Peach (1 medium)	

Fruits are **simple carbohydrates** because they contain fruit sugar. But because fruits contain a lot of water, fiber, and many important vitamins and minerals, they are not absorbed as quickly into your bloodstream as the simple-sugar sweets mentioned earlier and don't cause a quick rise and fall in blood sugar. Fruits are a rich source of vitamin C as well as vitamin A, potassium, and fiber. **Vitamin C** helps maintain body tissues, fights infections, promotes healing, and keeps your immune system healthy. **It is important to eat at least one fruit (or vegetable) high in vitamin C each day. Some foods high in vitamin C include papayas, oranges, grapefruit, cantaloupe, mangos, strawberries, red bell peppers, broccoli, and tomatoes.**

TIPS:

- Keep the fruit bowl full of fruits such as bananas, apples, oranges, apricots, and grapes for healthy snacking.
- Eat fresh fruit for dessert instead of highly processed sugary foods.
- Add fruit to your cereal in the morning.
- Freeze grapes, berries, and bananas for a frozen treat.

Dairy
(Milk, Yogurt, & Cheese)
• **3-4 servings per day** • **Approximately 90 calories per serving** • **Amounts listed are one serving size**

Cheese, hard (1 oz.) Evaporated skim milk (½ cup) Ice cream, non-fat, low-fat (½ cup) Milk, non-fat, skim, 1%, 2% (1 cup)	Non-fat dry milk (⅓ cup) Soy milk, with calcium, low-fat (1 cup) Tofu, with calcium (8 oz.) Yogurt, non-fat, low-fat (1 cup)

Dairy products are a rich source of **calcium** which is necessary for normal growth and development and for building strong bones and teeth. Because calcium is such an important nutrient for your baby, Mother Nature makes sure you always have enough calcium in your breast milk, even if you are not getting enough in your own diet. However, if you are lacking calcium in your diet, the needed calcium for your breast milk is taken from the supply stored in your own bones. **Dairy products high in calcium include milk, cheese, and yogurt. But you can also get calcium from nondairy sources such as turnip and mustard greens, fish with bones (salmon, sardines), broccoli, pinto beans, and corn tortillas as well as calcium-fortified cereals, tofu, and orange juice.**

TIPS:

- Start your day with dairy: have milk and cereal, yogurt with fruit, or a yogurt smoothie for breakfast.
- Add shredded cheese to soups, salads, casseroles, baked potatoes, and vegetables.
- Eat vegetables and fruits with yogurt dips.
- Make calcium-rich foods a snack-time choice—cheese cubes, yogurt, milk, frozen yogurt, or low-fat pudding.

Protein	
(Meat, Poultry, Fish, Dry Beans, Eggs)	
• **4 servings per day** • **Approximately 110–160 calories per serving** • **Amounts listed are one serving size**	
Beans, lentils, peas, cooked (1 cup) Beef, pork, poultry, cooked (2 oz.) Cheese, hard (2 oz.) Cottage cheese (1 cup) Eggs (2)	Luncheon meat (2 oz.) Peanut butter (2 tbs.) Fish (2 oz.) Tofu (1 cup) Shellfish, cooked (4 oz.)

Protein provides your body with iron, zinc, B vitamins and, amino acids, the building blocks that build, repair, and maintain your body tissues. **Since your body is not able to store protein as it does some other nutrients, you need to eat some protein-rich foods every day, preferably at every meal.** Moderate to low-fat protein sources such as lean meats, poultry, fish, and legumes are your best choices. Additionally, protein-rich foods provide you with iron. **Iron** is important for new mothers because it is helps to replace the iron stores lost during pregnancy. **Iron comes in two dietary forms: (1) animal sources such as red meat, beef liver, pork, chicken, egg yolks, fish, and shellfish; and (2) plant sources such as spinach, beans, dried fruit, pumpkin seeds, peanut butter, and soybeans. You can also find iron in fortified breakfast cereals and other iron-enriched grain products.** The iron from animal sources is better absorbed by your body than the iron from plant sources. To further increase iron absorption, eat foods or drink juices high in vitamin C at the same time you eat foods high in iron. Anemia can result if you don't get enough iron in your diet, which can make you feel weak, tired, and in poor health.

TIPS:

- Use mostly cooking methods that add little or no fat—broil, grill, roast, stew or steam rather than fry.
- Choose lean cuts of meats—round and loin cuts of beef, and loin cuts of pork and lamb. Look for extra-lean ground beef and low-fat lunch meats.
- Add legumes—beans, peas, and lentils—to tacos, burritos, soups, salads, stews, pasta sauces, and stir-fries.
- Try to eat seafood several times per week. It has less fat than meat or poultry, and contains omega 3 fatty acids, which may help protect you from heart disease.
- Use tofu, which is made from soybeans, in soups, casseroles, stir-fries, and other dishes.

Fats
• **4–8 servings per day** • **Approximately 45 calories per serving** • **Amounts listed are one serving size**

Avocado (1/8) Butter (1 tsp.) Bacon (1 slice) Cream cheese (1 tbs.) Half and half (2 tbs.) Margarine (1 tsp.)	Mayonnaise (1 tsp.) Nuts (2 tbs.) Oil (1 tsp.) Salad dressing (1 tbs.) Sour cream (2 tbs.)

Fats are an important part of a healthy diet and are also a necessary ingredient in breast milk. Fats provide your body with essential fatty acids that give you energy and help your body absorb fat-soluble vitamins such as A, D, E, and K. The fats contained in foods also help satisfy your hunger by making you feel full after eating. **Choose mostly unsaturated fats such as canola, nut, and olive oils, since they are healthier for you than hydrogenated vegetable oils (trans fats) and saturated fats found in animal products.** Use fats and oils sparingly, since they are all high in calories.

TIPS:

- Eat fewer processed foods such as packaged snacks and baked goods, since most contain hydrogenated vegetable oils (trans fats). These trans fats are linked to heart disease. Check the ingredient labels.
- Eat less saturated fats, which are found in animal products. Saturated fats are linked to heart disease and certain types of cancers and can raise blood cholesterol levels.
- Go easy on salad dressings, cream cheese, sour cream, and mayonnaise, since they are all high in saturated fats and calories. Try low-fat or fat-free versions.
- Eat nuts more often. They may be high in calories, but they are also high in nutrients and good (unsaturated) fats—and they tend to satisfy your hunger longer.

Fluids
• **Eight 8-oz. glasses per day** • **0 calories per serving** • **Amounts listed are one serving size**

Herbal tea (8 oz.) Mineral water (8 oz.)	Non-caloric beverage (8 oz.) Water (8 oz.)

Most nursing mothers notice an increase in thirst and automatically drink more water or other fluids. Try to drink at least eight 8-ounce glasses of fluid each day to keep up your milk supply. Water is a key nutrient and is required for many body functions. Water transports nutrients and oxygen to your cells, regulates your body temperature, aids in metabolism, and eliminates body waste. If you become constipated and have dark, strong-smelling urine, it is a sign that you are not getting enough fluids.

TIPS:

- Drink a large glass of water or a healthy beverage before breastfeeding.
- Add fruit juice or a squeezed lemon to sparkling water.
- You can also satisfy your need for fluids by drinking fruit juices, vegetable juices, yogurt drinks, and milk, but keep in mind that they do contain calories.

Combination Food Items

A slice of bread or a piece of fruit are easy to put into a food group. But where do pizza, cheeseburgers, and tacos fit in? It's easy to decide if you start with the main ingredient. Combination foods are made with several ingredients. Every combination food can be broken down into two or more food groups—even foods from different cultures—if you know the main ingredient. The following food exchange list[1] breaks down some of the most common combination food items into food group servings. This list will help you record your food intake in the "Nursing Mother's Daily Nutrition Checklist" beginning on PAGE 84. If a food is not on the list, just find the food closest to it. You don't have to be exact; approximations are fine.

Combination Food Items	
Food	**Food Exchange Value**
Burrito, beef or chicken (1)	2 grain, 1 protein, 2 fat
Casserole, tuna noodle (1 cup)	2 grain, 1 protein, 2 fat
Cheeseburger, beef (1 single)	2 grain, 1 protein, 2 fat
Chicken nuggets (6 pieces)	1 grain, 1 protein, 2 fat
Chicken sandwich, crispy (1)	3½ grain, 1 protein, 2 fat
Chicken sandwich, grilled (1)	2½ grain, 1½ protein, 1 fat
Chili with meat and beans (1 cup)	2 grain, 1 protein, 2 fat
Chow mein, beef, with noodles (1 cup)	2½ grain, 1 protein, 1 fat
Clam chowder, New England (1 cup)	1½ grain, 2 fat
Corn bread (2-oz. piece)	1 grain, 1 fat
Corn dog (1)	4 grain, ½ protein, 3 fat
Croissant (1 small)	1 grain, 2 fat
Enchilada, beef or chicken and cheese (1)	2 grain, 1 protein, 3 fat
Fajita, beef or chicken (1)	2 grain, 1 protein, 2 fat
Fish sandwich with tarter sauce (1)	3 grain, ½ protein, 4 fat
French fries (1 regular order)	2 grain, 2 fat
Hamburger, beef (1 single)	2 grain, 1 protein, 1 fat
Hot dog with bun (1)	1 grain, ½ protein, 2 fat
Lasagna (1 cup)	2 grain, 1 protein, 2 fat
Macaroni and cheese (1 cup)	2 grain, 1 protein, 2 fat
Pizza, cheese (¼ of 10-inch pizza)	2 grain, 1 protein, 2 fat
Pizza, combination (¼ of 10-inch pizza)	2 grain, 1 protein, 3 fat
Potato salad (½ cup)	1 grain, 2 fat
Quiche Lorraine (⅛ pie)	1 grain, 1½ protein, 4 fat
Soup, chicken noodle or vegetable beef (1 cup)	1 grain, 1 fat
Soup, cream (1 cup)	1 grain, 2 fat
Spaghetti with meat sauce (1 cup)	2 grain, 1 protein, 2 fat
Taco, beef or chicken, hard shell (1)	2 grain, 1 protein, 2 fat
Tostada, beef or chicken (1)	2 grain, ½ protein, 2 fat

[1]*Adapted from the U.S. Exchange Lists for Meal Planning devised by the American Diabetes Association and The American Dietetic Association*

Snack Foods, Desserts, and Alcoholic Beverages

The following food exchange list[2] breaks down some of the most common snack foods, desserts, and alcoholic beverages into food group servings. This list will help you occasionally include these foods in your eating plan—and continue to stay on track. However, when choosing these items, moderation is key, since most are high in fat and calories and/or highly processed and low in nutrients. Use this list to help you record your food intake in the "Nursing Mother's Daily Nutrition Checklist" beginning on PAGE 84.

Snack Foods, Desserts, and Alcoholic Beverages	
Food	**Food Exchange Value**
Beer (12 oz.)	3 fat
Beer, light (12 oz.)	2 fat
Brownie (1 small)	1 grain, 1 fat
Cake, angel food (1/12 of cake)	2 grain
Cake, chocolate, iced (1/12 of cake)	2½ grain, 2 fat
Cheese crackers (20)	1 grain, 1 fat
Cheesecake (1/12 of cake)	1½ grain, 4 fat
Cheese puffs (1 oz.)	1 grain, 2 fat
Chips, potato (1 oz.)	1 grain, 2 fat
Chips, tortilla (1 oz.)	1 grain, 2 fat
Cola or other flavored soda (8 oz.)	2 grain
Cookie, chocolate chip (1 medium)	1 ½ grain, 1 fat
Danish pastry, fruit filled (1)	3 grain, 3 fat
Doughnut, glazed or cake (1)	1½ grain, 2 fat
Granola bar (1)	1 grain, 1 fat
Gummy Bears (10 small)	2 grain
Ice cream, regular (½ cup)	1 grain, 1 fat
Jam or jelly (1 tbs.)	1 grain
M&M's plain (1 bag)	2 grain, 2 fat
M&M's with peanuts (1 bag)	2 grain, 3 fat
Milk chocolate bar (1.6 oz.)	2 grain, 3 fat
Milk shake, vanilla (medium)	4 grain, 1 fat
Nutri-grain Bar (1)	1½ grain, 1 fat
Pie, fruit, 2 crust (1/6)	3 grain, 2 fat
Pop-Tart pastry (1)	2½ grain, 1 fat
Pudding, regular or tapioca (½ cup)	2 grain, 1 fat
Reese's Peanut Butter Cups (2)	1½ grain, 3 fat
Ritz Crackers (10)	1 grain, 2 fat
Snickers Bar (1)	3 grain, 3 fat
Starburst Fruit Chews (6)	3 grain, 1 fat
Sun Chips (1 oz.)	1 grain, 1 fat
Tootsie Rolls (7 bite-size)	2 grain
Trail mix (¼ cup)	1 grain, 2 fat
Wine, red or white (4 oz.)	2 fat
Yogurt, frozen (½ cup)	1 grain

[2]*Adapted from the U.S. Exchange Lists for Meal Planning devised by the American Diabetes Association and The American Dietetic Association.*

Free Food Items

The foods on the following list have less than 20 calories per serving and are considered "free foods." When you eat these foods, you do **not** have to check off a box in the "Nursing Mother's Daily Nutrition Checklist." Foods that do not have a serving size listed next to them can be eaten as often as you like. However, foods with a serving size listed should be limited to 3 servings per day.

Free Food Items	
Bouillon, broth, consommé	Parsley
Catsup (1 tbs.)	Pickles, dill (1½ large)
Cream cheese, fat-free (1 tbs.)	Radishes
Garlic	Relish
Gelatin, sugar-free	Salad dressing, fat-free (2 tbs.)
Herbs and spices, fresh or dried	Salsa (¼ cup)
Horseradish	Sour cream, fat-free (1 tbs.)
Jam or jelly, low-sugar or light (2 tsp.)	Soy sauce
Lemon, lime	Sugar substitutes
Margarine, fat-free (4 tbs.)	Syrup, sugar-free (2 tbs.)
Mayonnaise, fat-free (1 tbs.)	Tabasco, hot pepper sauce
Miracle Whip, fat-free (1 tbs.)	Taco sauce (1 tbs.)
Mustard	Vinegar
Non-stick cooking spray	Worcestershire sauce

Fast Foods the Healthy Way

Although most fast foods are high in fat, sugar, and calories, they can still be a part of a healthy diet. You can continue to eat your favorite fast foods—cheeseburgers, pizza, milk shakes, and French fries—as long as your day is balanced with healthier lower fat and lower calorie foods. The following tips can help you make healthy food choices when visiting fast food restaurants.

TIPS:

- Just say "no" to *combo* and *super-size meals*—or get one meal and share it. Some of these meals have over 2,000 calories—a whole day's worth of calories!
- Order a regular-size meal (regular burger, fries, and milk or juice) which has less than half the calories of a combo or super-size meal.
- Better yet, order a *kid's meal* for a better value in price and calories!
- **Choose these more often:** grilled chicken or fish sandwiches, thin-crust pizza, vegetable wraps, green salads, baked potatoes, and low-fat frozen yogurt.
- **Choose these less often:** hamburgers with sauces, breaded and fried chicken or fish sandwiches, French fries, potato chips, milk shakes, and super-size soft drinks.

Sample Menu

As a new mother, you don't have a lot of extra time or energy to prepare fancy meals and snacks or follow a complicated eating plan. The table on the following page will show you a quick and easy sample menu for a nursing mother eating 1,800 calories per day. To make mealtimes easier, find recipes that have only a few ingredients and are easy to prepare. When you cook, double the recipe and save half for another meal. **The key to healthy eating is to eat mostly whole foods in their most natural state (whole grains, vegetables, and fruits) and go easy on the high-fat, highly processed, and sugary foods.**

Sample Menu For a Balanced Diet 1,800 Calories		
Meal	**Sample Food**	**Food Exchange Value**
BREAKFAST	Bran cereal, fortified (¾ cup) Low-fat milk (1 cup) Banana Orange juice (½ cup)	1 grain *(folic acid)* 1 dairy 1 fruit 1 fruit *(vitamin C)*
SNACK	Celery sticks (1 cup) Peanut butter (2 tbs.)	1 vegetable 1 protein *(iron)*
LUNCH	Cheeseburger Green Salad Salad dressing (1 tbs.) Low-fat milk (1 cup)	2 grain, 1 protein *(iron)*, 2 fat 1 vegetable 1 fat 1 dairy
SNACK	Pineapple chunks (1 cup) Cottage cheese (1 cup)	1 fruit 1 protein
DINNER	Tuna (2 oz.) with tomato (1 cup) Mayonnaise (1 tsp.) Brown rice (⅔ cup) Broccoli (½ cup) with melted cheese (1 oz.) Fresh cantaloupe (1 cup)	1 protein, 1 vegetable 1 fat 2 grain 1 vegetable, 1 dairy 1 fruit *(vitamin A)*
SNACK	Angel food cake Low-fat ice cream (½ cup)	2 grain 1 dairy
1,800 Total Calories: Grains = 7; Vegetables = 4; Fruits = 4; Dairy = 3; Protein = 4; Fats = 4		

Dietary Supplements

If you follow this plan, you will be eating a balanced diet that includes a variety of foods and all the vitamins and minerals you need while breastfeeding. However, some nursing mothers choose to continue taking their prenatal vitamins for the first few months of breastfeeding as nutritional insurance. If you are not getting enough iron in your diet, you may need iron supplements to replace the iron stores lost during pregnancy. Also, if your diet is restricted or you are vegetarian, dietary supplements may be recommended. However, before taking any dietary supplements, consult your health care provider or a nutritionist for the proper recommendations and dosage, since some supplements taken in excess can be dangerous.

Foods That Can Sometimes Cause a Reaction

Babies are happily breastfed all over the world while their mothers eat a wide variety of foods. You do not have to limit your diet in any way, unless you find that a particular food you are eating is causing a problem for your baby. This mostly occurs in sensitive babies who have a family history of allergies. Just remember that babies can be fussy and have gas just because they do, not necessarily because of something you ate or drank. The key is to tune into your baby. What affects your baby may be different from what affects another baby. For example, if your baby is fussy, has gas, a rash, or diarrhea 4 to 6 hours after you have eaten a grilled-cheese sandwich, a yogurt, and a glass of milk, he may be allergic to cow's milk products. In fact, the most common food sensitivity in nursing babies is to proteins found in cow's milk. Other foods that may cause a reaction are soy, wheat, fish, corn, and eggs. Some foods may cause gas, such as cabbage, broccoli, cauliflower, Brussels sprouts, and dried beans. Foods that are highly acidic such as oranges and tomatoes, and sometimes nuts and chocolate, may also bother your baby.

It usually takes about 4 to 6 hours for a food to affect your breast milk. If you believe something you are eating or drinking may be causing your baby discomfort, stop eating the food for about a week to see if the symptoms disappear. After a few weeks, you can try to adding the foods back into your diet, one by one, to see whether it continues to bother your baby after nursing. You may just need to avoid the foods temporarily, as most babies with food sensitivities usually outgrow them by 3 months of age. However, if you are finding it necessary to avoid certain food groups (such as dairy foods, citrus fruits, or wheat products), you may need to consult a nutritionist to help you plan an appropriate diet to make sure you are getting all the nutrients you need.

Caffeine

It is best to limit or avoid caffeine while you are breastfeeding. Even though only a small amount of caffeine passes into breast milk, it may build up in your baby's system and could cause irritability, nervousness, and wakefulness. Some nursing mothers are able to drink moderate amounts of caffeine each day (no more than the amount found in three 8-ounce cups of coffee) without it causing a problem. But if caffeine seems to be affecting your baby, or if you are having problems sleeping, it is best to avoid caffeine altogether. Caffeine is found in coffee, tea, colas, and chocolate. Since coffee and other caffeinated beverages are diuretics that pull water from your body, it is important to drink an extra ounce of water for every ounce of caffeine you consume. In addition, coffee in large amounts seems to affect iron absorption in both mother and baby.

Exercise

During the first 6 weeks postpartum your focus should be on developing a successful breastfeeding relationship with your baby and recovering from childbirth. But once you are feeling good and have your doctor's approval, you may begin an appropriate physical activity. Waiting at least 3 weeks postpartum before exercising is usually recommended after a normal vaginal delivery. If you had a cesarean delivery, most doctors recommend waiting at least 6 weeks postpartum before starting any type of exercise program. If you exercised regularly before and during your pregnancy, take care to ease yourself back into your usual exercise routine. If you didn't exercise before or during your pregnancy, it's even more important to start out slowly.

Walking

Walking is a perfect way to begin your postpartum exercise program. Taking walks with your baby will raise your spirits and remind you that there is life going on around you! You can start by walking with your baby in a baby carrier, and when he gets heavier you can put him in a baby stroller. Try to walk for at least 30 minutes, 3 times per week, at a pace that feels comfortable. Walking burns calories, tones your muscles, increases you metabolism, and helps control your appetite. You can gradually increase your pace to get your heart rate up. Listen to your body and it will tell you how active you can be during the early weeks. Now is a good time to start a regular routine of exercise so that it becomes a natural part of your family's life.

The Nursing Mother's Daily Nutrition Checklist

Sometimes new mothers are so busy with the new baby during the early days that they forget to eat! The **"Nursing Mother's Daily Nutrition Checklist"** on the following pages will help you get all the nutrition you need for the first week and help you get off to the right start. Use the daily check-off boxes to record your food group servings and fluid intake. There is also space to record your weight and exercise. By recording your food group servings and fluid intake after each meal and snack, you will easily be able to see where you are with your diet each day. If you get off track, just pick up where you left off and start again. Remember, you don't have to eat perfectly every single day. Balancing what you eat over several days is really what counts—not what you eat in a single meal or single day. You don't even have to change your regular eating pattern. You may eat three meals and three snacks or several mini meals per day, depending on your hunger level and your lifestyle. Start out slowly with small goals, such as eating more vegetables and fruits, having a better breakfast, or switching to whole-grain breads. Just do the best you can each day. Remember, all foods fit into a healthy eating plan. **Choose the foods that you love and that fit into your own lifestyle, but just remember that the key to healthy eating is to eat *mostly* whole foods in their most natural state (whole grains, vegetables, and fruits) and go easy on the high-fat, highly processed, and sugary foods. Bon appétit, Mom!**

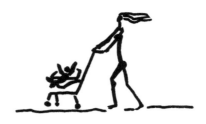

NURSING MOTHER'S DAILY NUTRITION CHECKLIST

DATE:

FOOD GROUP	DAILY SERVINGS	SERVING SUGGESTIONS
GRAINS **(7–12 servings)**	1 ☐ _____ 2 ☐ _____ 3 ☐ _____ 4 ☐ _____ 5 ☐ _____ 6 ☐ _____ 7 ☐ _____ 8 ☐ _____ 9 ☐ _____ 10 ☐ _____ 11 ☐ _____ 12 ☐ _____	Beans, peas, lentils, corn, cooked (½ cup) Bread, whole-grain, white, sliced (1) Breadsticks, 4-inch (2) Bun, hot dog, hamburger (½) Cereal, fortified, cold (¾ cup) Cereal, fortified, hot (½ cup) Couscous, polenta, cooked (⅓ cup) Crackers, pretzels (¾ oz.) Dinner roll (1) English muffin, bagel (½) Graham crackers (3 squares) Pasta, whole grain, white, cooked (½ cup) Popcorn, popped, fat-free (3 cups) Potato, baked (1 small) Potato, mashed (½ cup) Rice, risotto, cooked (⅓ cup) Rice cakes (2) Squash, pumpkin (1 cup) Sweet potato, yam (½ cup) Tortilla, pita, 6-inch (½) Waffle, pancakes, low-fat (1) Wheat germ (3 tbs.)
VEGETABLES **(4 servings)**	1 ☐ _____ 2 ☐ _____ 3 ☐ _____ 4 ☐ _____	Artichokes, asparagus, bean sprouts, beets, bok choy, broccoli, Brussels sprouts, cabbage, carrots, cauliflower, celery, cucumber, eggplant, green beans, jicama, kale, leeks, mushrooms, mustard greens, okra, onions, peppers, radishes, snow peas, spinach, tomatoes, turnip greens, turnips, water chestnuts, zucchini (1 cup raw, ½ cup cooked, ½ cup juice)
FRUITS **(4 servings)**	1 ☐ _____ 2 ☐ _____ 3 ☐ _____ 4 ☐ _____	Apple, banana, kiwi, peach, pear, orange (1) Apricots (4) Berries, all types (1 cup) Cantaloupe, melon, pineapple (1 cup) Cherries, grapes (12 large) Fruit juice (½ cup) Fruit nectar, dried fruit (¼ cup) Grapefruit, mango, papaya (½) Nectarines, plums, tangerines (2)
DAIRY **(3–4 servings)**	1 ☐ _____ 2 ☐ _____ 3 ☐ _____ 4 ☐ _____	Cheese, hard (1 oz.) Evaporated skim milk (½ cup) Ice cream, non-fat, low-fat (½ cup) Milk, non-fat, skim, 1%, 2% (1 cup) Non-fat dry milk (⅓ cup) Soy milk, with calcium, low-fat (1 cup) Tofu, with calcium (8 oz.) Yogurt, non-fat, low-fat (1 cup)
PROTEIN **(4 servings)**	1 ☐ _____ 2 ☐ _____ 3 ☐ _____ 4 ☐ _____	Beans, peas, lentils, cooked (1 cup) Beef, pork, poultry, fish, cooked (2 oz.) Cheese, hard (2 oz.) Cottage cheese, tofu (1 cup) Eggs (2) Luncheon meat (2 oz.) Peanut butter (2 tbs.) Shellfish, cooked (4 oz.)
FATS **(4–8 servings)**	1☐ 2☐ 3☐ 4☐ 5☐ 6☐ 7☐ 8☐	Avocado (⅛) Bacon (1 slice) Butter, margarine, mayonnaise, oil (1 tsp.) Cream cheese, salad dressing (1 tbs.) Sour cream, half and half, nuts (2 tbs.)
FLUID **(8 servings)**	1☐ 2☐ 3☐ 4☐ 5☐ 6☐ 7☐ 8☐	Herbal tea (8 oz.) Mineral water (8 oz.) Non-caloric beverage (8 oz.) Water (8 oz.)
WEIGHT	_____	**TOTAL POUNDS LOST** _____
EXERCISE	_____	**MINUTES** _____

84

NURSING MOTHER'S DAILY NUTRITION CHECKLIST

DATE:

FOOD GROUP	DAILY SERVINGS	SERVING SUGGESTIONS
GRAINS (7–12 servings)	1 ☐ _____ 2 ☐ _____ 3 ☐ _____ 4 ☐ _____ 5 ☐ _____ 6 ☐ _____ 7 ☐ _____ 8 ☐ _____ 9 ☐ _____ 10 ☐ _____ 11 ☐ _____ 12 ☐ _____	Beans, peas, lentils, corn, cooked (½ cup) Bread, whole-grain, white, sliced (1) Breadsticks, 4-inch (2) Bun, hot dog, hamburger (½) Cereal, fortified, cold (¾ cup) Cereal, fortified, hot (½ cup) Couscous, polenta, cooked (⅓ cup) Crackers, pretzels (¾ oz.) Dinner roll (1) English muffin, bagel (½) Graham crackers (3 squares) Pasta, whole grain, white, cooked (½ cup) Popcorn, popped, fat-free (3 cups) Potato, baked (1 small) Potato, mashed (½ cup) Rice, risotto, cooked (⅓ cup) Rice cakes (2) Squash, pumpkin (1 cup) Sweet potato, yam (½ cup) Tortilla, pita, 6-inch (½) Waffle, pancakes, low-fat (1) Wheat germ (3 tbs.)
VEGETABLES (4 servings)	1 ☐ _____ 2 ☐ _____ 3 ☐ _____ 4 ☐ _____	Artichokes, asparagus, bean sprouts, beets, bok choy, broccoli, Brussels sprouts, cabbage, carrots, cauliflower, celery, cucumber, eggplant, green beans, jicama, kale, leeks, mushrooms, mustard greens, okra, onions, peppers, radishes, snow peas, spinach, tomatoes, turnip greens, turnips, water chestnuts, zucchini (1 cup raw, ½ cup cooked, ½ cup juice)
FRUITS (4 servings)	1 ☐ _____ 2 ☐ _____ 3 ☐ _____ 4 ☐ _____	Apple, banana, kiwi, peach, pear, orange (1) Apricots (4) Berries, all types (1 cup) Cantaloupe, melon, pineapple (1 cup) Cherries, grapes (12 large) Fruit juice (½ cup) Fruit nectar, dried fruit (¼ cup) Grapefruit, mango, papaya (½) Nectarines, plums, tangerines (2)
DAIRY (3–4 servings)	1 ☐ _____ 2 ☐ _____ 3 ☐ _____ 4 ☐ _____	Cheese, hard (1 oz.) Evaporated skim milk (½ cup) Ice cream, non-fat, low-fat (½ cup) Milk, non-fat, skim, 1%, 2% (1 cup) Non-fat dry milk (⅓ cup) Soy milk, with calcium, low-fat (1 cup) Tofu, with calcium (8 oz.) Yogurt, non-fat, low-fat (1 cup)
PROTEIN (4 servings)	1 ☐ _____ 2 ☐ _____ 3 ☐ _____ 4 ☐ _____	Beans, peas, lentils, cooked (1 cup) Beef, pork, poultry, fish, cooked (2 oz.) Cheese, hard (2 oz.) Cottage cheese, tofu (1 cup) Eggs (2) Luncheon meat (2 oz.) Peanut butter (2 tbs.) Shellfish, cooked (4 oz.)
FATS (4–8 servings)	1☐ 2☐ 3☐ 4☐ 5☐ 6☐ 7☐ 8☐	Avocado (⅛) Bacon (1 slice) Butter, margarine, mayonnaise, oil (1 tsp.) Cream cheese, salad dressing (1 tbs.) Sour cream, half and half, nuts (2 tbs.)
FLUID (8 servings)	1☐ 2☐ 3☐ 4☐ 5☐ 6☐ 7☐ 8☐	Herbal tea (8 oz.) Mineral water (8 oz.) Non-caloric beverage (8 oz.) Water (8 oz.)
WEIGHT	_____	**TOTAL POUNDS LOST** _____
EXERCISE	_____	**MINUTES** _____

NURSING MOTHER'S DAILY NUTRITION CHECKLIST

DATE:

FOOD GROUP	DAILY SERVINGS	SERVING SUGGESTIONS
GRAINS **(7–12 servings)**	1 ☐ _____ 2 ☐ _____ 3 ☐ _____ 4 ☐ _____ 5 ☐ _____ 6 ☐ _____ 7 ☐ _____ 8 ☐ _____ 9 ☐ _____ 10 ☐ _____ 11 ☐ _____ 12 ☐ _____	Beans, peas, lentils, corn, cooked (½ cup) Bread, whole-grain, white, sliced (1) Breadsticks, 4-inch (2) Bun, hot dog, hamburger (½) Cereal, fortified, cold (¾ cup) Cereal, fortified, hot (½ cup) Couscous, polenta, cooked (⅓ cup) Crackers, pretzels (¾ oz.) Dinner roll (1) English muffin, bagel (½) Graham crackers (3 squares) Pasta, whole grain, white, cooked (½ cup) Popcorn, popped, fat-free (3 cups) Potato, baked (1 small) Potato, mashed (½ cup) Rice, risotto, cooked (⅓ cup) Rice cakes (2) Squash, pumpkin (1 cup) Sweet potato, yam (½ cup) Tortilla, pita, 6-inch (½) Waffle, pancakes, low-fat (1) Wheat germ (3 tbs.)
VEGETABLES **(4 servings)**	1 ☐ _____ 2 ☐ _____ 3 ☐ _____ 4 ☐ _____	Artichokes, asparagus, bean sprouts, beets, bok choy, broccoli, Brussels sprouts, cabbage, carrots, cauliflower, celery, cucumber, eggplant, green beans, jicama, kale, leeks, mushrooms, mustard greens, okra, onions, peppers, radishes, snow peas, spinach, tomatoes, turnip greens, turnips, water chestnuts, zucchini (1 cup raw, ½ cup cooked, ½ cup juice)
FRUITS **(4 servings)**	1 ☐ _____ 2 ☐ _____ 3 ☐ _____ 4 ☐ _____	Apple, banana, kiwi, peach, pear, orange (1) Apricots (4) Berries, all types (1 cup) Cantaloupe, melon, pineapple (1 cup) Cherries, grapes (12 large) Fruit juice (½ cup) Fruit nectar, dried fruit (¼ cup) Grapefruit, mango, papaya (½) Nectarines, plums, tangerines (2)
DAIRY **(3–4 servings)**	1 ☐ _____ 2 ☐ _____ 3 ☐ _____ 4 ☐ _____	Cheese, hard (1 oz.) Evaporated skim milk (½ cup) Ice cream, non-fat, low-fat (½ cup) Milk, non-fat, skim, 1%, 2% (1 cup) Non-fat dry milk (⅓ cup) Soy milk, with calcium, low-fat (1 cup) Tofu, with calcium (8 oz.) Yogurt, non-fat, low-fat (1 cup)
PROTEIN **(4 servings)**	1 ☐ _____ 2 ☐ _____ 3 ☐ _____ 4 ☐ _____	Beans, peas, lentils, cooked (1 cup) Beef, pork, poultry, fish, cooked (2 oz.) Cheese, hard (2 oz.) Cottage cheese, tofu (1 cup) Eggs (2) Luncheon meat (2 oz.) Peanut butter (2 tbs.) Shellfish, cooked (4 oz.)
FATS **(4–8 servings)**	1☐ 2☐ 3☐ 4☐ 5☐ 6☐ 7☐ 8☐	Avocado (⅛) Bacon (1 slice) Butter, margarine, mayonnaise, oil (1 tsp.) Cream cheese, salad dressing (1 tbs.) Sour cream, half and half, nuts (2 tbs.)
FLUID **(8 servings)**	1☐ 2☐ 3☐ 4☐ 5☐ 6☐ 7☐ 8☐	Herbal tea (8 oz.) Mineral water (8 oz.) Non-caloric beverage (8 oz.) Water (8 oz.)
WEIGHT	_____	**TOTAL POUNDS LOST** _____
EXERCISE	_____	**MINUTES** _____

NURSING MOTHER'S DAILY NUTRITION CHECKLIST

DATE:

FOOD GROUP	DAILY SERVINGS	SERVING SUGGESTIONS
GRAINS (7–12 servings)	1 ☐ _____ 2 ☐ _____ 3 ☐ _____ 4 ☐ _____ 5 ☐ _____ 6 ☐ _____ 7 ☐ _____ 8 ☐ _____ 9 ☐ _____ 10 ☐ _____ 11 ☐ _____ 12 ☐ _____	Beans, peas, lentils, corn, cooked (½ cup) Bread, whole-grain, white, sliced (1) Breadsticks, 4-inch (2) Bun, hot dog, hamburger (½) Cereal, fortified, cold (¾ cup) Cereal, fortified, hot (½ cup) Couscous, polenta, cooked (⅓ cup) Crackers, pretzels (¾ oz.) Dinner roll (1) English muffin, bagel (½) Graham crackers (3 squares) Pasta, whole grain, white, cooked (½ cup) Popcorn, popped, fat-free (3 cups) Potato, baked (1 small) Potato, mashed (½ cup) Rice, risotto, cooked (⅓ cup) Rice cakes (2) Squash, pumpkin (1 cup) Sweet potato, yam (½ cup) Tortilla, pita, 6-inch (½) Waffle, pancakes, low-fat (1) Wheat germ (3 tbs.)
VEGETABLES (4 servings)	1 ☐ _____ 2 ☐ _____ 3 ☐ _____ 4 ☐ _____	Artichokes, asparagus, bean sprouts, beets, bok choy, broccoli, Brussels sprouts, cabbage, carrots, cauliflower, celery, cucumber, eggplant, green beans, jicama, kale, leeks, mushrooms, mustard greens, okra, onions, peppers, radishes, snow peas, spinach, tomatoes, turnip greens, turnips, water chestnuts, zucchini (1 cup raw, ½ cup cooked, ½ cup juice)
FRUITS (4 servings)	1 ☐ _____ 2 ☐ _____ 3 ☐ _____ 4 ☐ _____	Apple, banana, kiwi, peach, pear, orange (1) Apricots (4) Berries, all types (1 cup) Cantaloupe, melon, pineapple (1 cup) Cherries, grapes (12 large) Fruit juice (½ cup) Fruit nectar, dried fruit (¼ cup) Grapefruit, mango, papaya (½) Nectarines, plums, tangerines (2)
DAIRY (3–4 servings)	1 ☐ _____ 2 ☐ _____ 3 ☐ _____ 4 ☐ _____	Cheese, hard (1 oz.) Evaporated skim milk (½ cup) Ice cream, non-fat, low-fat (½ cup) Milk, non-fat, skim, 1%, 2% (1 cup) Non-fat dry milk (⅓ cup) Soy milk, with calcium, low-fat (1 cup) Tofu, with calcium (8 oz.) Yogurt, non-fat, low-fat (1 cup)
PROTEIN (4 servings)	1 ☐ _____ 2 ☐ _____ 3 ☐ _____ 4 ☐ _____	Beans, peas, lentils, cooked (1 cup) Beef, pork, poultry, fish, cooked (2 oz.) Cheese, hard (2 oz.) Cottage cheese, tofu (1 cup) Eggs (2) Luncheon meat (2 oz.) Peanut butter (2 tbs.) Shellfish, cooked (4 oz.)
FATS (4–8 servings)	1☐ 2☐ 3☐ 4☐ 5☐ 6☐ 7☐ 8☐	Avocado (⅛) Bacon (1 slice) Butter, margarine, mayonnaise, oil (1 tsp.) Cream cheese, salad dressing (1 tbs.) Sour cream, half and half, nuts (2 tbs.)
FLUID (8 servings)	1☐ 2☐ 3☐ 4☐ 5☐ 6☐ 7☐ 8☐	Herbal tea (8 oz.) Mineral water (8 oz.) Non-caloric beverage (8 oz.) Water (8 oz.)
WEIGHT	_____	**TOTAL POUNDS LOST** _____
EXERCISE	_____	**MINUTES** _____

NURSING MOTHER'S DAILY NUTRITION CHECKLIST

DATE:

FOOD GROUP	DAILY SERVINGS	SERVING SUGGESTIONS
GRAINS **(7–12 servings)**	1 ☐ _____ 2 ☐ _____ 3 ☐ _____ 4 ☐ _____ 5 ☐ _____ 6 ☐ _____ 7 ☐ _____ 8 ☐ _____ 9 ☐ _____ 10 ☐ _____ 11 ☐ _____ 12 ☐ _____	Beans, peas, lentils, corn, cooked (½ cup) Bread, whole-grain, white, sliced (1) Breadsticks, 4-inch (2) Bun, hot dog, hamburger (½) Cereal, fortified, cold (¾ cup) Cereal, fortified, hot (½ cup) Couscous, polenta, cooked (⅓ cup) Crackers, pretzels (¾ oz.) Dinner roll (1) English muffin, bagel (½) Graham crackers (3 squares) Pasta, whole grain, white, cooked (½ cup) Popcorn, popped, fat-free (3 cups) Potato, baked (1 small) Potato, mashed (½ cup) Rice, risotto, cooked (⅓ cup) Rice cakes (2) Squash, pumpkin (1 cup) Sweet potato, yam (½ cup) Tortilla, pita, 6-inch (½) Waffle, pancakes, low-fat (1) Wheat germ (3 tbs.)
VEGETABLES **(4 servings)**	1 ☐ _____ 2 ☐ _____ 3 ☐ _____ 4 ☐ _____	Artichokes, asparagus, bean sprouts, beets, bok choy, broccoli, Brussels sprouts, cabbage, carrots, cauliflower, celery, cucumber, eggplant, green beans, jicama, kale, leeks, mushrooms, mustard greens, okra, onions, peppers, radishes, snow peas, spinach, tomatoes, turnip greens, turnips, water chestnuts, zucchini (1 cup raw, ½ cup cooked, ½ cup juice)
FRUITS **(4 servings)**	1 ☐ _____ 2 ☐ _____ 3 ☐ _____ 4 ☐ _____	Apple, banana, kiwi, peach, pear, orange (1) Apricots (4) Berries, all types (1 cup) Cantaloupe, melon, pineapple (1 cup) Cherries, grapes (12 large) Fruit juice (½ cup) Fruit nectar, dried fruit (¼ cup) Grapefruit, mango, papaya (½) Nectarines, plums, tangerines (2)
DAIRY **(3–4 servings)**	1 ☐ _____ 2 ☐ _____ 3 ☐ _____ 4 ☐ _____	Cheese, hard (1 oz.) Evaporated skim milk (½ cup) Ice cream, non-fat, low-fat (½ cup) Milk, non-fat, skim, 1%, 2% (1 cup) Non-fat dry milk (⅓ cup) Soy milk, with calcium, low-fat (1 cup) Tofu, with calcium (8 oz.) Yogurt, non-fat, low-fat (1 cup)
PROTEIN **(4 servings)**	1 ☐ _____ 2 ☐ _____ 3 ☐ _____ 4 ☐ _____	Beans, peas, lentils, cooked (1 cup) Beef, pork, poultry, fish, cooked (2 oz.) Cheese, hard (2 oz.) Cottage cheese, tofu (1 cup) Eggs (2) Luncheon meat (2 oz.) Peanut butter (2 tbs.) Shellfish, cooked (4 oz.)
FATS **(4–8 servings)**	1☐ 2☐ 3☐ 4☐ 5☐ 6☐ 7☐ 8☐	Avocado (⅛) Bacon (1 slice) Butter, margarine, mayonnaise, oil (1 tsp.) Cream cheese, salad dressing (1 tbs.) Sour cream, half and half, nuts (2 tbs.)
FLUID **(8 servings)**	1☐ 2☐ 3☐ 4☐ 5☐ 6☐ 7☐ 8☐	Herbal tea (8 oz.) Mineral water (8 oz.) Non-caloric beverage (8 oz.) Water (8 oz.)
WEIGHT	_____	**TOTAL POUNDS LOST** _____
EXERCISE	_____	**MINUTES** _____

NURSING MOTHER'S DAILY NUTRITION CHECKLIST

DATE:

FOOD GROUP	DAILY SERVINGS	SERVING SUGGESTIONS
GRAINS **(7–12 servings)**	1 ☐ _____ 2 ☐ _____ 3 ☐ _____ 4 ☐ _____ 5 ☐ _____ 6 ☐ _____ 7 ☐ _____ 8 ☐ _____ 9 ☐ _____ 10 ☐ _____ 11 ☐ _____ 12 ☐ _____	Beans, peas, lentils, corn, cooked (½ cup) Bread, whole-grain, white, sliced (1) Breadsticks, 4-inch (2) Bun, hot dog, hamburger (½) Cereal, fortified, cold (¾ cup) Cereal, fortified, hot (½ cup) Couscous, polenta, cooked (⅓ cup) Crackers, pretzels (¾ oz.) Dinner roll (1) English muffin, bagel (½) Graham crackers (3 squares) Pasta, whole grain, white, cooked (½ cup) Popcorn, popped, fat-free (3 cups) Potato, baked (1 small) Potato, mashed (½ cup) Rice, risotto, cooked (⅓ cup) Rice cakes (2) Squash, pumpkin (1 cup) Sweet potato, yam (½ cup) Tortilla, pita, 6-inch (½) Waffle, pancakes, low-fat (1) Wheat germ (3 tbs.)
VEGETABLES **(4 servings)**	1 ☐ _____ 2 ☐ _____ 3 ☐ _____ 4 ☐ _____	Artichokes, asparagus, bean sprouts, beets, bok choy, broccoli, Brussels sprouts, cabbage, carrots, cauliflower, celery, cucumber, eggplant, green beans, jicama, kale, leeks, mushrooms, mustard greens, okra, onions, peppers, radishes, snow peas, spinach, tomatoes, turnip greens, turnips, water chestnuts, zucchini (1 cup raw, ½ cup cooked, ½ cup juice)
FRUITS **(4 servings)**	1 ☐ _____ 2 ☐ _____ 3 ☐ _____ 4 ☐ _____	Apple, banana, kiwi, peach, pear, orange (1) Apricots (4) Berries, all types (1 cup) Cantaloupe, melon, pineapple (1 cup) Cherries, grapes (12 large) Fruit juice (½ cup) Fruit nectar, dried fruit (¼ cup) Grapefruit, mango, papaya (½) Nectarines, plums, tangerines (2)
DAIRY **(3–4 servings)**	1 ☐ _____ 2 ☐ _____ 3 ☐ _____ 4 ☐ _____	Cheese, hard (1 oz.) Evaporated skim milk (½ cup) Ice cream, non-fat, low-fat (½ cup) Milk, non-fat, skim, 1%, 2% (1 cup) Non-fat dry milk (⅓ cup) Soy milk, with calcium, low-fat (1 cup) Tofu, with calcium (8 oz.) Yogurt, non-fat, low-fat (1 cup)
PROTEIN **(4 servings)**	1 ☐ _____ 2 ☐ _____ 3 ☐ _____ 4 ☐ _____	Beans, peas, lentils, cooked (1 cup) Beef, pork, poultry, fish, cooked (2 oz.) Cheese, hard (2 oz.) Cottage cheese, tofu (1 cup) Eggs (2) Luncheon meat (2 oz.) Peanut butter (2 tbs.) Shellfish, cooked (4 oz.)
FATS **(4–8 servings)**	1☐ 2☐ 3☐ 4☐ 5☐ 6☐ 7☐ 8☐	Avocado (⅛) Bacon (1 slice) Butter, margarine, mayonnaise, oil (1 tsp.) Cream cheese, salad dressing (1 tbs.) Sour cream, half and half, nuts (2 tbs.)
FLUID **(8 servings)**	1☐ 2☐ 3☐ 4☐ 5☐ 6☐ 7☐ 8☐	Herbal tea (8 oz.) Mineral water (8 oz.) Non-caloric beverage (8 oz.) Water (8 oz.)
WEIGHT	_____	**TOTAL POUNDS LOST** _____
EXERCISE	_____	**MINUTES** _____

89

NURSING MOTHER'S DAILY NUTRITION CHECKLIST

DATE:

FOOD GROUP	DAILY SERVINGS	SERVING SUGGESTIONS
GRAINS **(7–12 servings)**	1 ☐ _____ 2 ☐ _____ 3 ☐ _____ 4 ☐ _____ 5 ☐ _____ 6 ☐ _____ 7 ☐ _____ 8 ☐ _____ 9 ☐ _____ 10 ☐ _____ 11 ☐ _____ 12 ☐ _____	Beans, peas, lentils, corn, cooked (½ cup) Bread, whole-grain, white, sliced (1) Breadsticks, 4-inch (2) Bun, hot dog, hamburger (½) Cereal, fortified, cold (¾ cup) Cereal, fortified, hot (½ cup) Couscous, polenta, cooked (⅓ cup) Crackers, pretzels (¾ oz.) Dinner roll (1) English muffin, bagel (½) Graham crackers (3 squares) Pasta, whole grain, white, cooked (½ cup) Popcorn, popped, fat-free (3 cups) Potato, baked (1 small) Potato, mashed (½ cup) Rice, risotto, cooked (⅓ cup) Rice cakes (2) Squash, pumpkin (1 cup) Sweet potato, yam (½ cup) Tortilla, pita, 6-inch (½) Waffle, pancakes, low-fat (1) Wheat germ (3 tbs.)
VEGETABLES **(4 servings)**	1 ☐ _____ 2 ☐ _____ 3 ☐ _____ 4 ☐ _____	Artichokes, asparagus, bean sprouts, beets, bok choy, broccoli, Brussels sprouts, cabbage, carrots, cauliflower, celery, cucumber, eggplant, green beans, jicama, kale, leeks, mushrooms, mustard greens, okra, onions, peppers, radishes, snow peas, spinach, tomatoes, turnip greens, turnips, water chestnuts, zucchini (1 cup raw, ½ cup cooked, ½ cup juice)
FRUITS **(4 servings)**	1 ☐ _____ 2 ☐ _____ 3 ☐ _____ 4 ☐ _____	Apple, banana, kiwi, peach, pear, orange (1) Apricots (4) Berries, all types (1 cup) Cantaloupe, melon, pineapple (1 cup) Cherries, grapes (12 large) Fruit juice (½ cup) Fruit nectar, dried fruit (¼ cup) Grapefruit, mango, papaya (½) Nectarines, plums, tangerines (2)
DAIRY **(3–4 servings)**	1 ☐ _____ 2 ☐ _____ 3 ☐ _____ 4 ☐ _____	Cheese, hard (1 oz.) Evaporated skim milk (½ cup) Ice cream, non-fat, low-fat (½ cup) Milk, non-fat, skim, 1%, 2% (1 cup) Non-fat dry milk (⅓ cup) Soy milk, with calcium, low-fat (1 cup) Tofu, with calcium (8 oz.) Yogurt, non-fat, low-fat (1 cup)
PROTEIN **(4 servings)**	1 ☐ _____ 2 ☐ _____ 3 ☐ _____ 4 ☐ _____	Beans, peas, lentils, cooked (1 cup) Beef, pork, poultry, fish, cooked (2 oz.) Cheese, hard (2 oz.) Cottage cheese, tofu (1 cup) Eggs (2) Luncheon meat (2 oz.) Peanut butter (2 tbs.) Shellfish, cooked (4 oz.)
FATS **(4–8 servings)**	1☐ 2☐ 3☐ 4☐ 5☐ 6☐ 7☐ 8☐	Avocado (⅛) Bacon (1 slice) Butter, margarine, mayonnaise, oil (1 tsp.) Cream cheese, salad dressing (1 tbs.) Sour cream, half and half, nuts (2 tbs.)
FLUID **(8 servings)**	1☐ 2☐ 3☐ 4☐ 5☐ 6☐ 7☐ 8☐	Herbal tea (8 oz.) Mineral water (8 oz.) Non-caloric beverage (8 oz.) Water (8 oz.)
WEIGHT	_____	**TOTAL POUNDS LOST** _____
EXERCISE	_____	**MINUTES** _____

CHAPTER 7

Starting Solid Foods and Weaning

Weaning is the word used to describe the period when your child becomes less and less dependent on your breast milk for nourishment and then stops breastfeeding completely. Weaning begins as soon as you give your baby something besides your breast milk and ends when you are no longer nursing at all. The important thing about weaning is that you do it gradually. There may be some strong emotions attached to weaning, since it is one of the first steps a child takes in becoming independent from his mother. Sometimes weaning may cause a mother to have feelings of sadness. This is usually due to the sudden decrease in *prolactin*, the mothering hormone, and the realization that breastfeeding is coming to an end. These feelings are normal and usually pass with time.

When to Start Solid Foods

It is recommended that you wait until your baby is about 6 months old before offering him solid foods. If you introduce solid foods too early, it can interfere with breastfeeding and the immune benefits of your breast milk. Some foods may also promote allergies. Most babies will let you know when they are ready to start eating solid foods. When your child is ready, he may seem hungry after nursing and become very interested in the foods you are eating. He may even try to grab the food off your plate! **When solid foods are introduced, they should be *added* to the breast milk diet, *not replace it*.**

Solid foods give your baby additional calories, protein, iron, minerals, and other nutrients, as well as new tastes and textures. Giving your baby solid foods begins the gradual shift to an adult diet of table foods. Iron-fortified, single-grain infant cereals, such as rice cereal, make an excellent first food because they are easily digested and less likely to cause allergies. Also, breastfed babies need other sources of iron in their diets after about 6 months, and these iron-fortified infant cereals will meet this requirement. Infant cereals should be mixed with expressed breast milk rather than cow's milk. (Giving cow's milk to babies under one year of age is not recommended because it can cause allergies.) Begin by mixing the cereal with your breast milk to a very thin consistency, and then gradually thicken the texture as your baby gets used to solids. It's best to offer solid foods in the afternoon or evening, after your baby has already had a good amount of breast milk. You can also start offering your baby liquids from a cup, such as water or unsweetened fruit juice with a little water added. Fruit juices should only be offered to your baby about once a day. Giving babies too much fruit juice can affect their health because it decreases their appetites for wholesome foods.

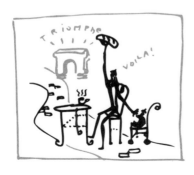

When starting solid foods, most experts recommend giving your baby a single new food at a time for several days to make sure he can tolerate it. After infant cereals, you can offer your baby strained fruits or vegetables. You can start by mixing the infant cereal with a fruit such as applesauce, bananas, pears, or peaches, or a vegetable such as carrots, sweet potatoes, squash, or peas instead of breast milk. Then you can move on to strained meats, which are high in protein, iron, vitamins, and minerals. Chicken and turkey make good first meat choices. As your baby gets older, you can offer him bite-size pieces of fruits, vegetables, and meats, as well as finger foods such as cheese cubes, baby teething cookies, and ring cereals.

Suggestions for Weaning

The question of when to wean your child is a personal decision that will depend on both you and your child. Some mothers choose to wean after only a few months of breastfeeding, while others let their child decide when he is ready to stop nursing. Some babies simply lose interest in the breast between 9 and 12 months of age and prefer a cup or solid foods to breastfeeding. Sometimes weaning may be necessary when a mother and baby are separated for a long period of time. The reasons for weaning (when and why) are different for every mother and baby pair. But the most important thing about weaning is to do it slowly. Weaning too quickly can cause breast discomfort.

When weaning happens naturally it is usually a gradual process. Typically at about 9 months of age, your baby may become less interested in the breast. Sometimes he may not want to nurse and would rather drink from a bottle or cup. At other times you may miss a feeding and realize that your baby didn't mind at all. Before long you are breastfeeding only once or twice per day. Your milk supply slowly lessens until eventually you aren't breastfeeding at all. This can take from a few weeks to a few months. Here are some suggestions for weaning your baby:

- Begin by replacing one feeding at a time with solid foods or liquids, depending on your baby's age. This feeding should be the one that he is least interested in, usually during the day.
- After a few days, replace another feeding.
- Keep this up every few days until he is weaned completely.
- Keep your baby busy with other activities such as reading stories, playing games, going for walks, or other distractions.
- Your milk production will gradually decrease, but you may need to hand express or pump just enough milk to relieve fullness until your breasts stop making milk completely.
- If it is necessary to wean suddenly, you can use ice packs to reduce engorgement and relieve breast discomfort.
- Give your baby lots of extra love and attention during the weaning period. It will give him confidence as he becomes more independent.

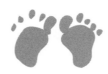

CHAPTER 8

Working and Breastfeeding

Planning Ahead

Even if you have to return to work, it doesn't mean you have to stop breastfeeding. Many mothers who work outside the home have successfully continued to breastfeed their babies while working part-time or full-time jobs. Knowing that your baby will continue to get the health benefits of your breast milk while you are apart will make it worth the effort. Breastfed babies have healthier immune systems and are less likely to catch the many viruses that go around child care centers. Breastfeeding also helps you keep that special feeling of closeness you have with your baby while you are away. The longer you can put off going back to work, the better for you and your baby. If possible, try to wait until your baby is at least 6 weeks old before returning to work. This will give you a chance to bond with your baby and build up your milk supply. Going back to work and breastfeeding does take some planning. This chapter will help you be successful at combining working and breastfeeding.

Talk to Your Employer

No matter what type of job you have, your breaks and your lunch hour should be yours to spend as you choose. Why not use this time to pump your breast milk and continue to give your baby the best nutrition possible? Before you return to work talk to your employer about your plan to combine working and breastfeeding. Explain why breastfeeding is important to you, why pumping is necessary, and how you plan to fit pumping into your work schedule. Also let your employer know that breastfed infants do not get sick as often as formula-fed infants, so you will miss fewer days of work to take care of a sick baby.

Fortunately, more and more employers are realizing the important role women have in the workforce today and are making it easier for breastfeeding mothers to return to work. Many employers realize that if they support breastfeeding, they will have lower health care costs and happier employees, which in the long run will save them money. Some employers even provide "breast-pumping breaks" and "lactation rooms" where mothers can pump.

Let your employer know that you will need to take at least two or three 30-minute breaks during the day to pump your breast milk. This will keep your milk flowing and provide you with milk to give to your baby at a later time. Ask where you can pump at work, and make sure it is a private, clean, and quiet area. Also check to see if there is a refrigerator to store the milk. If one is not available, you can bring in a small

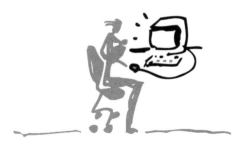

cooler with ice packs. If it is possible, discuss changing your work schedule temporarily. Ask about working part-time or flexible hours for the first few months. Or, if your child care provider is close to your work, you may be able to arrange to breastfeed your baby during your breaks.

Prepare to Pump Before You Go Back to Work

It is best to start pumping and collecting your breast milk about 2 weeks before you plan to go back to work. This will give you a chance to practice using the breast pump and build up a good supply of pumped breast milk for your first week. It will also give your baby some time to get used to taking a bottle. This may be difficult at first. You may need to have someone else give him the bottle of expressed breast milk, because when he sees you he thinks of breastfeeding. Here are some tips for preparing to go back to work:

- Start pumping your breast milk 2 weeks before going back to work. Pump about 1 hour after your first feeding in the morning and 2 or 3 times during the day between feedings.
- Store the breast milk in small amounts, 2 to 4 ounces per storage container. Label the containers with your baby's name, the date collected, and the amount.
- Introduce your baby to the bottle about 2 weeks before you go back to work. Experiment with different types of nipples to find one your baby likes.
- You may need to have someone else feed your baby the bottle of expressed breast milk, if he does not want to take it from you.

Choosing Child Care

Choosing a child care provider for your baby is an important decision. Knowing that your baby is in good hands while you are apart will make going back to work a little easier. Ideally, begin looking for child care while you are still pregnant. Look for someone you trust and feel comfortable with and who supports breastfeeding. This person should be able to handle feeding your baby bottled breast milk according to your instructions. Here are some tips for choosing a child care provider:

- It may help to find a child care provider close to your work. If you are able to leave work, it will make it easier for you to go to your baby to nurse, or you can have him brought to you.
- Pay an unannounced visit to the child care provider at least once before making your decision.
- Once you have made a decision, visit the child care provider with your baby before returning to work so your baby can become familiar with the new faces and surroundings.
- Let the child care provider know that you would like your baby to be held while he is being fed and picked up when he cries or fusses.
- Once you are back at work, check in often. If you are not happy with how things are going, don't be afraid to change child care providers—follow your instincts.

Returning to Work

Once you are back at work, make a plan for the times you will express your breast milk. You will need to pump at the times you would normally breastfeed your baby. This is usually about every 3 hours. The average time it takes to pump is about 30 minutes, or less if you are using a double pump. Following this schedule will ensure that you keep up your milk supply to meet your baby's needs. Pumping on schedule will also help with engorgement and leaking breasts. Here are some tips for returning to work:

- Get everything ready the night before: pack the diaper bag, have the bottles of breast milk ready in the refrigerator, pick out your outfits, pack your lunch, and make sure your breast pump is clean and ready.
- Nurse your baby first thing in the morning so you can get ready with fewer interruptions.
- Plan to nurse your baby just before leaving him with the child care provider.
- Leave your child care provider enough milk for the day, usually about three or four 4-ounce bottles for a newborn (and a little extra, just in case). The amount will increase as your baby grows.
- Babies eat about 2½ ounces of breast milk each day for every pound they weigh. (So a 10-pound baby would eat about 25 ounces of breast milk per day.)
- Start your first day back at work on a Wednesday for a shorter first week.
- While at work, pump your milk as often as you would nurse your baby (about every 3 hours for most mothers).
- Ask your child care provider to hold off feeding your baby close to pick-up time, so your baby will be ready to nurse when you arrive.
- Nurse your baby during the times you are together—when you get home, evenings, nighttime, and weekends.
- Talk to other working breastfeeding mothers for support and to share ideas.
- If working and pumping becomes too stressful, it doesn't have to be all or nothing. You can choose to give your baby formula while you are at work and nurse when you are together. Nursing part-time is better than not nursing at all. You may have to pump at work (just enough to relieve fullness) for a week or so, until your breasts adjust to not being emptied during the day.

Expressing Breast Milk

Whether you are going back to work or just need to express occasionally, you will want to be familiar with the different ways to express breast milk. How you remove the milk from your breasts, either manually or with a breast pump, will depend on the situation. Manual expression works well for engorgement and to soften the breasts just before a feeding. Breast pumps are recommended when you are returning to work or need to be separated from your baby for a period of time. A breast pump is also recommended if you have a premature or sick infant who is not able to take milk from your breasts, or when you need to increase your milk supply.

Learning to express your breast milk takes some time and practice. It usually takes about the same amount of time to express your breast milk as it does to breastfeed, unless you are using an automatic double breast pump, which is faster. Triggering the let-down reflex is important in order to express a good amount of breast milk. If you are having problems getting your milk to flow, you may find it helpful to look at a picture of your baby. You can also try applying a warm, moist towel to your breast and massaging. Try to clear your mind of stressful thoughts and make sure you are comfortable. Once your milk begins to flow, think about your baby.

Manual Expression

Expressing milk by hand is helpful in situations where you want to soften the breasts just before a feeding or relieve engorgement. Some mothers prefer the natural way of expressing breast milk and never have to buy a breast pump. To use this method, wash your hands thoroughly before you begin. Start by gently massaging your breast with your fingertips in an outward circular motion, from the chest wall toward the nipple. Then, form the letter "C" with your hand, placing your thumb on the top part of the areola and your four fingers underneath. Press straight back into the chest wall while squeezing your thumb and forefinger together. Continue this back-and-together motion until the milk begins to flow. It may take a few tries to get your hand positioned correctly so that the milk flows. Rotate your hand around the breast to reach all of the milk ducts. Continue until the flow stops. Avoid pinching or pulling on the breasts, as breast tissue is very delicate.

Using a Breast Pump

If you are planning to express your breast milk more than occasionally, a breast pump is recommended. Using a breast pump is a quick, efficient way to express your breast milk. When you first try to pump, you may get only a small amount of milk, just enough to cover the bottom of the container. However, do not become discouraged. It may take some time before your breasts become used to the suction of the breast pump. The key to successful pumping is to be comfortable and relaxed. Take a few minutes before each pumping session to unwind. Thinking about your baby or looking at his photograph may help get the milk flowing. If you are using the breast pump properly, you will soon see an increase in the amount of milk expressed, and pumping will become almost as natural as breastfeeding. Always read the manufacturer's instructions before using your breast pump.

How to Choose a Breast Pump

Deciding which breast pump is best for you will depend on how often you plan to pump your breast milk. There are several types of breast pumps on the market today. Breast pumps range in price, from under $50 (manual, some battery-operated, and smaller electric pumps) to over $200 (electric pumps that include a carrying case and other accessories). If you are only going to be away from your baby for a few hours a week, you can purchase a less expensive breast pump. However, if you are going back to work, it is worth using a good quality electric breast pump. You can usually rent a hospital-grade electric breast pump from a hospital lactation center or WIC clinic.

Manual Pumps. Manual pumps are portable and do not need a power source. However, to use a manual pump you must use both hands while pumping a piston or squeezing a lever repeatedly. Manual pumps are best for occasional short-term pumping.

Battery-operated Pumps. Battery-operated pumps are easier to use than manual pumps. They are inexpensive and only require one hand to operate. Since it is necessary to replace the batteries frequently, some are available with an AC electrical adapter.

Electric Pumps. Electric pumps are the fastest and most efficient type of breast pump and are best for long-term pumping. They are ideal for working mothers who need to pump more often. Electric pumps are very effective and comfortable to use. Better quality electric pumps have a built-in pressure cycle that is similar to the suction of a breast-feeding baby. There are several styles and sizes to choose from to meet your personal needs. Some electric breast pumps come with attachments that allow you to "double pump"—pump both breasts at the same time. Some may also come with battery packs, adapters, and other accessories.

Storing Breast Milk

You can store your expressed breast milk in plastic bags, plastic bottles, or glass containers designed specifically for storing breast milk. You will notice that the cream will separate and rise to the top of the container. This is normal because breast milk isn't *homogenized* (the process by which the milk fat is blended into the liquid). Breast milk may be safely stored by carefully following these steps:

1. Wash your hands thoroughly with soap and water.
2. Make sure all breast pump parts are clean and dry.
3. Pump or manually express your breast milk into a clean container.
4. Transfer the milk into a clean storage container.
5. Store breast milk in small amounts (2 to 4 ounces per container) for quicker thawing and to avoid waste.
6. If you are planning to freeze the milk, fill the container only ¾ full to allow room for it to expand.
7. Label the container with your baby's name, the date, and the amount.
8. Always use the oldest dated milk first.

Refrigeration. Breast milk that is not used right away can be kept safely at room temperature for up to 8 hours. However, refrigeration is recommended. Fresh breast milk can be stored in the refrigerator for up to 8 days. (If you are away from a refrigerator, it can be stored in an insulated cooler with ice packs for up to 24 hours.) Remove the sealed container of milk from the refrigerator just before a feeding and place it in a bowl of warm water, or hold the container under warm running water until it reaches room temperature. Never microwave breast milk, as it may destroy some of the natural immune properties and could heat unevenly, causing burns.

Freezing and defrosting. For longer storage, you can freeze your breast milk. Breast milk may be stored in a refrigerator freezer for up to 3 months or in a deep freezer for up to 6 months. Always place the breast milk containers in the coldest part of the freezer, away from the door.

To defrost:
1. Place the sealed container of frozen milk in a bowl of warm water, or hold the container under warm running water until it reaches room temperature.
2. Blend any cream that may have separated and risen to the top by swirling the container.
3. Test the milk on your wrist to see if it is warm enough for your baby.
4. Use thawed breast milk immediately after defrosting, or store it in the refrigerator and use it within 24 hours.
5. You can also thaw breast milk in the refrigerator as long as it is used within 24 hours.
6. Do not thaw frozen breast milk by letting it stand at room temperature.
7. Do not thaw frozen breast milk in a microwave oven.
8. Do not refreeze breast milk once it has been thawed.
9. Throw away any defrosted breast milk that is not used at a feeding.
10. Throw away any defrosted breast milk that smells or tastes sour.

Breast Milk Storage Recommendations Chart		
LOCATION	**TEMPERATURE**	**STORAGE TIME**
At room temperature	66°– 72°F (19°–22°C)	4 to 8 hours
In an insulated cooler with ice packs	60°F (15°C)	up to 24 hours
Refrigerator	32°– 39°F (0°– 4°C)	up to 8 days
Separate refrigerator freezer	temperature varies	up to 3 months
Deep freezer	0°F (-19°C)	up to 6 months

Traveling With Breast Milk

When transporting breast milk to use on outings away from home, it should be kept cold until it is ready to be fed to your baby. Use a small insulated cooler with ice packs to keep the milk cold during transport.

The
New Mother's
Journal

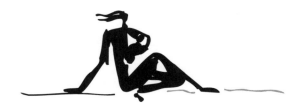

Baby's Birth Record

**Place baby's
newborn
photo here.**

Baby's Full Name _____

Date of Birth _____ Hair Color_____

Time of Arrival _____ Eye Color _____

Place of Birth_____ Weight _____

Doctor _____ Length _____

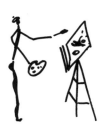

*Each time you look at your child you see something mysterious and contradictory—bits and
pieces of other people—grandparents, your mate, yourself, all captured
in a certain stance, a shape of the head, a look in the eyes, combined with something
very precious—a new human soul rich in individuality and possibility.*

—Joan Sutton

Childbirth Experience

That it will never come again is what makes life so sweet.
—Emily Dickinson

Writing about your childbirth experience can be a good way to help you adjust to motherhood. Writing down the details of your baby's birth will help you remember the events that took place. Later on, you and your child can look back at these memories and celebrate his or her birth. It is important to write about your childbirth experience while it is still fresh in your mind, because even an event as unforgettable as this does fade with time.

Where were you when you realized you were in labor? _____

_____

How did you know you were in labor? _____

_____

What time did you start having contractions? _____

Where was your partner when the contractions began? _____

_____

When did you tell your partner you were in labor? _____

_____

What was your partner's reaction? _____

_____

Who took you to the hospital? _____

_____

How long did it take you to get to the hospital and what time did you arrive?_____

_____

How did you feel when you arrived at the hospital? _____

_____

What helped you through the pain of labor? _____

_____

_____

How did your partner support you during labor? _____

_____

_____

Who was invited to attend the birth of your baby? _____

_____

_____

What memorable things happened during the labor and delivery? _____

_____

_____

How long did your labor last? _____

What emotions did you have when you first saw your baby?_____

_____

How did your partner react when he saw the baby for the first time? _____

_____

How did the people in the delivery room react to the birth? _____

_____

What is the first thing you noticed about your baby? _____

_____

Who does your baby look like? _____

_____

Who cut your baby's umbilical cord?_____

Were you able to hold your baby immediately after birth? _____

Did you nurse your baby immediately after birth? _____

_____

What was it like to nurse you baby for the first time? _____

_____

Who was the first person to visit you in the hospital after the birth? _____

_____

Who was the first person you called after the birth? _____

_____

How close to the due date was your baby born? _____

_____

How long was your hospital stay? _____

What was the weather like on the day your baby was born? _____

_____

What major events were in the news on the day your baby was born? _____

_____

_____

How do you feel about the whole experience of pregnancy and childbirth? _____

_____

_____

What do you want to someday tell your child about his entrance into the world?

_____

_____

_____

Idea Starters

We do not remember days, we remember moments.
—*Cesare Pavese*

Below is a list of questions to give you ideas of what to write about in your journal. You will be able to look at this journal with your child one day and you will be glad you took the time now to write down your memories.

1. How did you feel when you first brought your baby home?
2. Who was your baby's first visitor at home?
3. What was the reaction of your baby's grandparents when they saw the baby?
4. What was it like breastfeeding your baby during the first few days?
5. How does your baby let you know when he is hungry?
6. What has your breastfeeding experience been like?
7. Who gave you the most help in learning how to nurse your baby?
8. What is the biggest change now that you have a new baby in the house?
9. How has your relationship with your partner changed?
10. In what ways is your partner helping to make these first few days easier?
11. How does your partner help care for the baby?
12. In what new ways do you appreciate your partner?
13. What is the biggest surprise about your partner in his new role as father?
14. How do you feel when you see your partner caring for your baby?
15. When did your baby take his first bath?
16. What seems to make your baby happy?
17. When is your baby most cheerful during the day?
18. How does your baby like to be held, rocked, comforted, and entertained?
19. What gave you the biggest laugh since bringing your baby home?
20. What changes have you noticed in your baby since birth?
21. How has having your own child made you appreciate your own parents?
22. Have your feelings toward working outside the home changed?
23. What is the biggest surprise about having a baby?
24. What memories would you like to share with your child about his first days of life?

Date _____

_____

_____

_____

_____

_____

_____

_____

_____

_____

_____

_____

_____

_____

_____

_____

_____

_____

_____

_____

_____

_____

Where there is woman there is magic.
—Ntozake Shange

Date _____

_____

_____

_____

_____

_____

_____

_____

_____

_____

_____

_____

_____

_____

_____

_____

_____

_____

_____

_____

Let your heart guide you. It whispers, so listen closely.
—The Land Before Time

Date _____

_____

_____

_____

_____

_____

_____

_____

_____

_____

_____

_____

_____

_____

_____

_____

_____

_____

_____

_____

_____

_____

Look lovingly upon the present, for it holds the only things that are forever true.
—A Course In Miracles

Date _____

☀ _____

_____

_____

_____

_____

_____

_____

_____

_____

_____

_____

_____

_____

_____

_____

_____

_____

_____

Of all the rights of women, the greatest is to be a mother.
—*Lin Yu-tang*

Date _____

_____

_____

_____

_____

_____

_____

_____

_____

_____

_____

_____

_____

_____

_____

_____

_____

_____

_____

_____

_____

Other things may change us, but we start and end with family.
—Anthony Brandt

Date _____

_____

_____

_____

_____

_____

_____

_____

_____

_____

_____

_____

_____

_____

_____

_____

_____

_____

_____

_____

We ourselves feel that what we are doing is just a drop in the ocean.
But the ocean would be less because of that missing drop.
—Mother Teresa

Date _____

_____

_____

_____

_____

_____

_____

_____

_____

_____

_____

_____

_____

_____

_____

_____

_____

_____

_____

_____

_____

Nothing is permanent but change.
—Heraclitus

Where to Find Help

La Leche League International

1400 North Meacham Road
P.O. Box 4079
Schaumburg, IL 61068-4079
Phone: 1-800-La-Leche (1-800-525-3243) Weekdays, 9AM to 5PM Central Time
Fax: 1-847-519-0035
Website: www.lalecheleague.org

La Leche League International is a nonprofit organization founded in 1956 by a group of nursing mothers who wanted to help other mothers learn about breastfeeding. Today it is an internationally recognized authority on breastfeeding and offers mother-to-mother breastfeeding support. La Leche League Leaders hold meetings once a month all over the world to discuss breastfeeding topics and family related issues. They also have a Peer Counseling Program for nursing mothers. Peer Counselors are mothers who have nursed their babies and have been trained to help other mothers breastfeed. To find out the location of the nearest La Leche League meeting, to order a free catalog of breastfeeding books and products, or for answers to breastfeeding questions, call their 800 number or visit their Website.

Women, Infants, and Children (WIC)

USDA Food and Nutrition Services
3101 Park Center Drive
Alexandria, VA 22302
Website: www.fns.usda.gov/wic

The Supplemental Nutrition Program for Women, Infants, and Children, also known as WIC, provides nutritious foods, information on healthy eating, and health care referrals to pregnant and breastfeeding women and children up to age 5. WIC also encourages mothers to breastfeed and offers breastfeeding information and support. Mothers who breastfeed can participate longer in the WIC program and receive larger food packages than mothers who formula feed. Some WIC locations offer breast pump rentals and other breastfeeding accessories to help mothers breastfeed longer. Many WIC clinics also have Peer Counseling Programs. Peer Counselors are mothers who have nursed their babies and have been trained to help other mothers breastfeed. In order to qualify for WIC, you must be in need of additional nutritious foods to be healthy and meet certain income standards. To find the location of your nearest WIC clinic, you can call your local public health department or visit the Website listed above.

The National Women's Health Information Center
Breastfeeding Helpline

Phone: 1-800-994-WOMAN (800-994-9662) Weekdays, 9AM to 5PM Eastern Time
Phone: 1-888-220-5446 (TDD) for deaf and hearing impaired callers
Website: www.4woman.gov

The National Woman's Health Information Center (NWHIC) offers information on women's health. Recently, they have partnered with La Leche League International to train their Information Specialists so they can give new mothers the support they need to breastfeed. The Helpline, which operates in both English and Spanish, answers questions about common breastfeeding topics such as nursing positions and pumping and storing breast milk. They can also provide tips for working mothers who would like to continue breastfeeding, and offer suggestions for financial support. The Helpline is open to nursing mothers as well as their partners and families, prospective parents, health professionals, and institutions seeking to better educate new mothers about the benefits of breastfeeding. Ask about their free breastfeeding information packet.

International Lactation Consultant Association (ILCA)

1500 Sunday Drive, Suite 102
Raleigh, NC 27607
Phone: 1-919-861-5577
Website: www.ilca.org

The International Lactation Consultant Association (ILCA) can refer you to an experienced lactation consultant (IBCLC) in your area who has been certified by the International Board of Lactation Consultant Examiners. Certified lactation consultants work in hospitals, clinics, doctor's offices, and private practices helping mothers to breastfeed.

The American Dietetic Association (ADA)

120 South Riverside Plaza, Suite 2000
Chicago, IL 60606-6995
Phone: 1-800-366-1655 (Consumer Nutrition Information Line)
Website: www.eatright.org

This organization can help you find a nutritionist in your area and offers information on food and nutrition. Members of the ADA are nutritionists who have met stringent academic and professional requirements entitling them to put the letters R.D. (Registered Dietitian) after their names.

Index

A

After-pains, 66
Alcohol, 9–10, 79
Allergies
  cows milk products as cause, 48, 82, 91
  family history, 48, 81
  foods in mother's diet, 81–82
  formula as cause, 60
Alveoli, 20
American Academy of Pediatrics (AAP), 3
American Dietetic Association (ADA), 78–79,
  113
Antibodies
  in human milk, 4, 11, 22, 63
  to certain illnesses, 12
Areola, 5, 18, 20

B

Baby blues, 66
Baby's Birth Record, 100
Baby's Feeding and Diaper Log, 38–40
Battery-operated pumps, 97
Benefits, of breastfeeding, 2, 4, 11–13
Bilirubin, 22, 46
Biting, 49
Birth control pills, 10
Bottles
  avoiding nipple confusion, 19, 21, 45
  introducing, 19
  expressed breast milk, 5, 94, 97
Bowel movements
  as a sign of milk supply, 34–35
  constipation, 48
  diarrhea, 47
  frequency, 34, 37
  meconium, 30
  odor, 2, 34
  transitional stools, 34
Breast(s)
  basic care, 18
  engorged, 52–53
  fatty tissue, 6
  flat nipples, 17–18
  glandular tissue, 6, 17, 20
  infection (*See* Mastitis)
  inverted nipples, 17–18
  leaking, 53
  normal nipples, 17
  offering both, 32
  plugged ducts, 53–54
  preparing, 18

  size, 6
  surgery, 7, 17
Breast infection (*See* Mastitis)
Breast milk
  colostrum, 22
  composition, 4
  defrosting, 98
  expressing, 95–96
  foremilk, 32
  freezing, 97
  hindmilk, 32
  increasing supply, 56–57
  is baby "getting enough," 35
  let-down reflex, 20
  mature milk, 31
  nutritional deficiency in, 69
  production, 20
  refrigeration, 97
  storing, 97
  supply and demand, 19
Breast pumps
  battery operated, 97
  electric, 97
  how to choose, 96
  manual expression, 96
  manual pumps, 96
Breast shells, 18
Breastfeeding
  after a cesarean, 63
  benefits of, 2, 11
  breast preparation, 18
  duration (length of feedings), 28–29, 32
  first feeding, 22
  frequency (how often), 28–29, 32
  how breastfeeding works, 19
  how soon after delivery, 22
  in public, 41–42
  is baby "getting enough," 35
  laws, 43
  multiples, 64
  nutrition, 69–90
  positions, 26–28
  pregnancy and, 10
  premature baby, 63
  preparing for, 17–19
  sexuality and, 41
  working and, 11, 93
Breastfeeding Baby in Training, sign for hospital,
  23
Burping, 29

C

Cesarean, breastfeeding after, 63
Caffeine, 48, 82
Calcium, requirement for the nursing mother, 75
Calorie requirement for the nursing mother, 70
Candida albicans, 55

Childbirth Experience, 101
Child care, choosing, 94
Cluster feeding, 32–33
Clutch hold (*See* Football hold)
Colic, 48–49
Colostrum, 20, 22, 30, 31
Combination Food Items List, 78
Constipation
    in baby, 48
    in mother, 73
Contractions, uterine (*See* After-pains)
Cradle hold, 27
Cross cradle hold, 27

D

Dairy
    requirement for the nursing mother, 75
    causing a reaction in your baby, 82
Daily calorie requirement, 70
Daily food group servings, 72
Defrosting, of frozen breast milk, 97–98
Dehydration, signs of, 35–36
Depression, postpartum, 67
Diarrhea, 47
Diet, mother's, 69
Dietary supplements, 81
Drugs, 10
Ducts, plugged, 53–54

E

Elimination patterns, 33–34
Embarrassment, 5, 41
Emotional changes in mother, 66–67
Engorgement, 52-53
Episiotomy, 66
Exercise, 82–83
Explosive stool, 34
Expressing breast milk
    choosing a breast pump, 96–97
    manual expression, 96
    how to express, 95–97
    storing, 97
    traveling with breast milk, 98
    using a breast pump, 96

F

False alarms, recognizing, 57–58
Fats, requirement for the nursing mother, 77
Father, What to Expect as a Breastfeeding, 14–15
Fatty tissue, 6
Feeding(s)
    baby's first, 22
    duration (length of), 28, 32
    Feeding and Diaper Log, baby's, 38–40
    frequency (how often), 28, 32

    measuring, 28–29
    nighttime, 33
    signs of hunger, 29
Fever
    as a sign of mastitis, 55
    as warning sign in baby, 59
    as warning sign in mother, 58
Flat nipples, 17–18
Fluids, requirement for the nursing mother,
    77–78
Folic acid (folate), requirement for the nursing
    mother, 74
Food exchange lists, 72–80
Food Exchange System (U.S.), 71
Food group servings, determining mother's daily,
    72
Food Guide Pyranud (USDA), 71
Foods
    to limit or avoid while breastfeeding, 8–9, 82
    causing a reaction in baby, 81–82
Football hold, 28
Foremilk, 32
Formula, infant, 4, 7, 11–12
Free Food Items List, 80
Freezing, of breast milk, 97
Fruits, requirement for the nursing mother,
    74–75

G

Gastroesophageal reflux (GER), 47
Grains, requirement for the nursing mother, 73
Growth spurts, 34
Glandular tissue, 6, 17, 20

H

Hand expression (*See* Manual expression)
Hand pumps (*See* Manual pumps)
Hiccups, 29
Hindmilk, 32
Hunger cues in baby (*See* Signs of hunger)

I

Idea Starters, for New Mother's Journal, 104
Imprinting, 22
Increasing your milk supply, 56–57
International Board of Lactation Consultant
    Examiners (IBLCE), 113
Inverted nipples, 17–18
Iron, requirement for the nursing mother, 76

J

Jaundice
    abnormal (pathological), 46
    bilirubin, 46

checking for, 46
normal (physiologic), 46
phototherapy, 46
symptoms, 46
Jealousy
in partner, 7, 67

K

Keeping Track of Your Breastfeeding Baby, 37

L

La Leche League International, 18, 112
Lactation specialist, when to call, 58
Latch-on, 25–26
Leaking, 53
Let-down reflex, 20
Lip blisters, 46
Lochia, 65
Low milk supply, 56–57

M

Mammary glands, 20
Manual expression, 96
Manual pumps, 96
Mastitis, 55
Mature milk, 31
Meconium, 30
Medications, 10
Milk (*See* Breast milk)
Milk ducts, 20
Milk sinuses, 20
Milk-ejection reflex (*See* Let-down reflex)
Milk production, 20
Milk supply, increasing, 57
Montgomery glands, 20
Mother, What to Expect as a Breastfeeding, 13
Motherhood,
    adjusting to, 65
    emotional changes, 66–67
    physical changes, 65–66
    relationship changes, 67–68
Multiples, breastfeeding, 64

N

National Women's Health Information Center, 113
Nighttime feedings, 33
Nipple(s)
    care of, 18
    flat, 17–18
    inverted, 17–18
    normal, 17
    tenderness, 4, 41, 51
Nipple confusion, 45

Nipple shields, 18
New Mother's Journal, 99–111
Normal nipple, 17
Nursing Mother's Daily Nutrition Checklist, 83–90
Nursing strike, 49–50
Nutrition
    benefits of breast milk, 2, 4, 11–13
    for the nursing mother, 69–90

O

Offering both breasts, 32
Overview of Week 1, 37
Oxytocin, 20, 41, 53, 66

P

Pacifiers, 45
Phototherapy, 46
Physical changes, in mother, 65–66
Plugged ducts, 53–54
Positioning and latch-on, 25–28
Positions
    cradle hold, 27
    cross cradle hold, 27–28
    football hold, 28
    side-lying, 28
Postpartum blues (*See* Baby blues)
Postpartum depression, 66
Pregnancy and breastfeeding, 10
Premature baby, breastfeeding the, 63–64
Prenatal vitamins, 81
Projectile vomiting, 47
Prolactin, 20, 91
Protein, requirement for the nursing mother, 76
Pumping and storing breast milk (*See* Expressing breast milk)
Pyloric stenosis, 47

R

Refrigeration, of breast milk, 97
Relationship changes, in mother, 67–68
Returning to work, 93–95
Rooming-in, 21
Rooting reflex, 29

S

Sample menu, 81
Sexuality and breastfeeding, 41
Shields, nipple, 18
Side-lying position, 28
SIDS (*See* Sudden Infant Death Syndrome)
Signs of dehydration, in baby, 35–36
Signs of hunger, in baby, 29
Sitz bath, 66

Sleeping
  in bed with baby, 33
  nighttime feedings, 33
Sleepy baby
  switch nursing, 30
  waking, 29
Smoking, 9
Snack Foods, Desserts, and Alcoholic Beverages
  List, 79
Soiled diapers (*See* Bowel movements)
Solid foods, 91–92
Sore nipples, 51–52
Spitting up, 46–47
Spoiling baby, 5
Stenosis, pyloric, 47
Stools (*See* Bowel movements)
Sucking problems, 45
Sudden Infant Death Syndrome (SIDS), 2, 9, 12
Supplements, dietary, for the mother, 81
Supply and demand, 19
Switch nursing, 30

T

Thrush, 55–56
Tongue-tied, 45
Transitional stools, 34
Traveling with breast milk, 98
Twins, breastfeeding, 64

U

U.S. Department of Agriculture (USDA)
  Food Guide Pyramid, 71
U.S. Food Exchange System, 71
Urinary output
  as a sign of milk supply, 30, 34, 35, 37
  color, 30, 34, 35, 37
  normal for breastfed babies, 30, 34, 35, 37
Uterine contractions (*See* After-pains)

V

Vegetables, requirement for the nursing mother,
  74
Vitamin supplements (*See* Dietary supplements)
Vitamin A, requirement for the nursing mother,
  74
Vitamin C, requirement for the nursing mother,
  75
Vomiting
  as a warning sign, 47, 59
  projectile, 47
  pyloric stenosis, 47

W

Waking the sleepy baby, 29–30

Walking, 82–83
Warning signs, when to call a lactation specialist,
  58
Warning signs, when to call the doctor,
  for the baby, 59
  for the mother, 58–59
Water, requirements for the nursing mother, 77
Weaning, 92
Weight gain, in baby, 30
Weight loss
  in baby, 30
  in mother, 9, 69
Wet diapers (*See* Urinary output)
Where to find help, 112
Women, Infants, and Children (WIC), 19, 96, 112
Working and breastfeeding, 11, 93

Y

Yeast infection, as a sign of thrush, 55

About the Author

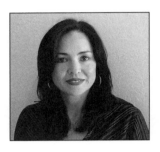

Elaine Moran is a former breastfeeding mother who became a Certified Lactation Counselor (CLC) after her two children were born. When she discovered that many of the problems she had while breastfeeding were preventable, she decided to write an uplifting, user-friendly breastfeeding guide to help all new mothers nurse their babies successfully—and avoid making the same mistakes. Elaine has a Bachelor of Arts degree in Psychology from California State University at Long Beach and a degree in Marketing from the Fashion Institute of Design and Merchandising in San Francisco. She is a volunteer counselor for the Nursing Mothers Counsel and a member of La Leche League International. Elaine has held various positions in her career including substitute teacher for the Pajaro Valley Unified School District, Merchandise Planner for Ross Department Stores, Weight Loss Counselor for Jenny Craig International, and Style Editor for CTB/McGraw-Hill. But being a mother has been her most challenging and rewarding career. Elaine lives in Northern California with her husband and two children. She nursed each of her children for their first year of life and looks back on those days with fond memories that she will always treasure.

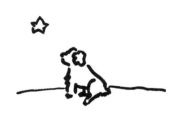